Gut Health Secrets

How Gut Health Affects Your Whole Body & Mind

Rachel Miner

Forward by Jessika Wagner, MD

Gut Health Secrets
How Gut Health Affects Your Whole Body & Mind
by Rachel Miner

Published by: Upper Shelf Reader
2122 W 1800 N #338
Clinton, Utah 84015 USA
Orders: 801-820-3799
uppershelfreader@gmail.com

Cover design and graphic artwork by Shaun Reid Miner

First Edition Copyright © 2019 Printed in the United States

ISBN: 978-0-9974624-1-8

Dedication

This book is dedicated to those who search
for answers to health issues knowing deep
inside there are answers to be found.

Contents

Forward

Why should you care about your gut and want to learn about these secrets? Because your gut is responsible for more than you realize. It is not just about digestion, nutrient absorption, and waste elimination.

I am a full time Pediatrician, mom of 4 little kids, and wife to an amazing guy. I am a food allergy mom. I am a Celiac disease mom and wife. You will find my full story in this book.

When I was in medical school over a decade ago, I learned about these basic functions of the gut. It was not until 2012 at a Continuing Medical Education Lecture that I started to hear more about gut health and the tremendous impact it has on our general health. Over the next few years I became more and more interested in gut health.

I learned that the gut plays an important role in lipid metabolism, insulin regulation, hormone production (including serotonin and melatonin), weight management, sleep, mood, energy, immune function, and even skin disorders.

Ultimately I learned, through study and personal experience with phenomenal supplementation and probiotics since 2016, that when you heal the gut, everything else starts to heal and life gets better!

Rachel Miner does a wonderful job laying out these 'secrets' in this book - things that are not well known but should be!

-Jessika Wagner, MD

Secret 1

Health: A Scale of 1 to 10

When I was five years old, I woke up one morning to find my eyes swollen shut. I thought I had gone blind. The reality was my eyes were glued shut from all the goop that came out of them during the night. I had developed allergies and my eyes gooped up from being around all the pollens in the air when I played outside. For a little five year old girl, it was both frightening and devastating to wake up and think I had gone blind.

During spring and summer months I would have to wake up and put warm cloths over my eyes until the goop came off enough for me to open up my eyes and see. I spent much of my time inside because just a small step out into nature would throw my health in such a tizzy. I would not be able to breathe, see, or resist the urge to scratch the rash on my body that appeared if I touched grass, weeds, or animals.

I was allergic to everything that had fur, and most everything growing outside that was green, from trees, to grasses and weeds. Grasses and horses had the worst effect on me, and I lived on an acre of horse property next to fields of farm land.

My siblings and neighbor friends being 'typical kids' made fun of the fact that the whites of my eyes would swell so dramatically with edema that it appeared my eyes were coming out of their sockets and kids called me 'The Weapon.' My brother told all of the neighbor kids that if they looked at me, they would go blind or die.

After enduring a few years of kid torture and miserable summers I was able to start getting allergy shots. Shots two times a weeks in both arms made life a little more bearable. Combined with shots, my mother took me to a Naturopath who prescribed homeopathic drops. Summers were still no fun, but I survived. I learned that I could play outside, but not sit on grass. I could be around animals, but not pet them. If I played outside for very long, I would come in and take a shower before bedtime to get all the pollen off me so I would not be as congested at night. My mother had to also put my pillow in the dryer before bed to kill all the allergens.

I usually slept poorly because breathing through my mouth made my mouth bone dry. I would have to drink water and then try to go back to sleep. Breathing through my nose was never on option because it was always stuffed.

In my early teens I developed depression. I would wonder why I just always felt sad. Some of the time I would think about taking a long rest to get away from the sadness. I fought with my parents and siblings and hated my life. What I never really understood was my life was really great and it was the depression following me around that was causing the sadness. I remember one time taking pills hoping it would take away the pain, only to wake up later to the same reality of life.

I have always been athletic. After years of gymnastics and riding my bike alongside my father who was a runner, I started running with him. I slowly increased the distance I ran each time and began to love it more and more. Distance running was my favorite. I loved the quiet alone time I had with myself to think and ponder on my runs.

Despite being a runner, I always had a high percentage of body fat. My high school coach would check our body fat percentage and made comments about me being a higher percentage of body fat than the other girls on the team. I would wonder if I 'exercised a little more,' would my body fat percentage decrease. So I increased my running to the point of exhausting my health in overexertion which almost landed me in the hospital and left me with severe health issues. The depression worsened and anemia, anxiety, bulimia and other 'girl' health issues arose. I learned to cope with the depression, anxiety, and bulimia by suppressing and hiding it from others.

Over the years I tried shots, pills, natural doctors, chiropractors, homeopathic treatments, supplements, oils and so much more. I never found answers or solutions to my health issues, but did find a few 'band aids' to help keep me in survival mode.

As a runner in college, I had a few years of peace from my allergies. This came from living in Hawaii with a tropical climate. I was also using a lot of natural remedies, colon cleanses, and educating myself on alternative holistic approaches to my health. The owner of the natural supplement store in town loved seeing my face because she knew she would be able to sell me 'the next best thing' every time I came to visit.

A few years later, after leaving the islands, getting married and having kids, my depression became worse. Fatigue, anxiety, and weight issues started to creep into my life along with constant headaches, sensitivity to light, stomach issues, sleepless nights, bowel issues, and feeling trapped. These symptoms were my 'new normal.' I thought I was a strong woman and never let anyone know the struggles I faced on a daily basis.

I really was not strong. My husband and kids suffered because I always had a black cloud that followed me throughout the day. I was not showing up in my life; I was just going through the motions.

I called it 'zombie-ing through life,' I got up, figured what it would take just to get to the end of the day, and then dread night time because that meant lying awake for hours before the next day would come and the cycle would start again. Many times, the black cloud almost won the best of me. Through lots of loving family, prayers, and guardian angels that watched over me constantly, I survived.

I was a silent sufferer. A silent sufferer is someone who suffers everything on their own never sharing what they are going through with anyone else. They put on a happy face and pretend life is great. I always wondered what other people would really think of me if they knew what I was struggling with. The trash talk in my head took the best of me for so many years.

After years of struggling, doctor visits, trying every 'new thing' to help me feel better, I was sick and tired of being sick and tired. I went to the doctor one more time to try to get help and that is when I had a scare with cancer.

This scare with cancer hit me like a ton of bricks. How could this be? How did I get here? What caused this? This pondering led me back to the roots I had studied so much about in my teenage and college years- natural alternatives for healing. I started researching more information on being healthy, and you know what it all led back to… gut health.

Gut health? Could that really have been the secret that no one told me all along? I had learned snippets about gut health over the years, but had never reached that 'aha' moment of how it was all related. Every problem, health issue, and struggle I had all lead back to the root cause of poor gut health. My gut had been out of whack since I was five years old (probably since birth) and it has wreaked havoc ever since.

As a teenager, I learned about Candida (yeast) from my mom. I took sugar control pills and tried cleanses. I would go with my mom to natural health food stores where we learned about muscle testing to see which supplements and nutrients our bodies needed. I even did research papers in college on homeopathic treatments and remedies. I just never put all of the pieces together, looking at it as one big puzzle connecting my whole body together.

After more research about gut health, I learned how all my symptoms were related. I learned that by adding in proper supplements I could start healing the gut. I researched natural supplements. I compared ingredients and the quality of nutrients in them. I found the right natural supplements for my body to start my healing process.

I combined these supplements with exercise and better eating. I was using everything as a tool leading me in the right direction for better health. I finally was able to find myself again and be the happy person I knew was inside of me, just trapped and waiting to get out. You know when you have an 'aha' moment and you wonder why you had never come up with that thought before. I had that 'aha' moment with gut health. I had been searching all those years and the answer was right before my eyes.

Yes, I am now on a much healthier path, but I wish I had found all this great information on gut health years ago. I know gut health is the secret to a better life, better health, and happiness that no one knows, or really cares to get educated on. People hear the term 'gut health' and the first thing that pops into their heads is to think about constipation and bloating. Yes, gut health does include those things, but it is so much more and I want everyone to realize how, if they just learned a little bit about gut health, they could have the power to feel so much better.

So Why 'Secrets?' Secrets are things kept unknown by others. Secrets are something we all want to be a part of. When you know a secret you are 'part of the club.' Think back to when you were a kid and everyone knew a secret but you. How did that make you feel? When you were finally included in the secret you felt powerful and now you were part of 'the club.' You were included.

I call these gut health secrets because it took me a lot of research, study, trial and error to find the gut health answers I was looking for. I felt like they were secrets that were being kept from me and I could have saved myself a lot of years of pain and suffering.

If I had known these secrets earlier in my life I could have treated symptoms by getting to the root of the cause of my health issues. I know gut health secrets are the missing link in most health issues.

By learning these secrets for yourself you will be included. You will be part of the club. You will be able to live life to the fullest. You will enjoy the journey you are on and share this knowledge with others who may be searching for answers to their own health problems. You can let them in on the secrets too.

You may be thinking that you just need to accept your life 'as is' because that is what happens as you get older, NO! You will learn here in this book that there are answers that can help you feel great again. It will give hope back to the hopeless and it will give health back to the sick.

This is why I care. This is why I will share all my gut health secrets with you. I do not want them to be secrets anymore.

Where to Start

Let me start with a little background. In the Renaissance time, bodies were painted with curves and rolls. These curves and rolls represented a 'healthy' person. A person who had meat on their bones in a time of survival was 'healthy.'

When fashion took over from survival, thinner was better. A person who was thin was considered 'healthy' and everyone strived for that.

People wanted to be thin and flat chested. They all wanted to be a flapper. Women would even bind their chests to have a thin appearance. That also began the era of all kinds of diet related health issues. Anorexia and bulimia began to emerge even more. This is when what we looked like became more important than how we felt and functioned.

On a scale of 1 to 10 where is your health? Who determines what those numbers on the scale represent? What do people consider to be good health? These are all questions that most people do not think about until their health takes a turn for the worse. An illness pops up or a diagnosis of a disease makes them take a step back and see where their health has taken them.

Thankfully we are beginning to come full circle in an age of understanding. The mind-body connection and how good nutrition and gut health affects our anxiety, depression and other health related issues and diseases.

Learning about gut health can take you on a journey of understanding the mind and body and what you can do to improve your health.

Gut Health

What is gut health anyway? You have heard the words and you probably made an assumption of what it means.

Starting from the mouth traveling all the way to the other end, where the waste comes out, everything in between and even around it is considered part of gut health. The digestive tract includes the mouth, esophagus, stomach, pancreas, liver, gallbladder, small intestine, colon, and rectum. Gut health also includes all of the microorganisms that live in and around our digestive tract. The microorganisms in and on our bodies are called the microbiome. The microbiome consists of bacteria, fungi, and viruses that all reside in, or on, our body. The microbiome is like a DNA for the gut.

For years, we thought of bacteria as organisms to avoid. It turns out our bodies are already loaded with trillions of bacteria. The bacteria in our microbiome help digest food and play an important role in our well-being.

The health of your gut is related to and affects all aspects of your body. We are coming to the realization that all of the functions in the body are related to each other. Gut health ties everything together. Through research we have learned our gut microbiome is tied to our probability of things like: diabetes, obesity, depression, and colon cancer. Just like the DNA of our bodies, our microbiome is unique to each individual, and no two people's microbiome are identical.

Over the years, as I went to doctors looking for answers, I would leave feeling frustrated. The doctors would only want to talk about one issue or one area of my body, because that is what he or she specialized in. I always wanted a doctor to address my whole body all together. I would take lists of everything wrong and come home frustrated after having only addressed one or two things on my list. I would think to myself how all my issues were related to one another. One thing going haywire in my body would lead to another and then another.

Now I know gut health is the secret. The gut health secret was the missing link. Gut health is what ties the body all together. The more I heal my gut the more healthier my body can be.

As you learn about the gut health secrets it will be helpful to put it into perspective of how it relates in personal situations. I have included stories of how improving gut health has positively impacted the health of everyday people. By hearing their stories you can relate how it would have a positive impact to improve your own health. Wherever your health is now the future can always be brighter than the past.

Emily, mother of four, and former teacher is the happiest person you will ever meet. She is a TV personality and cooking guest on Good Things Utah. She shares how survival mode had become her normal in life. I know mothers with kids of all ages can relate to her.

I remember waking up in the morning feeling like my bed covers weighed 1,000 pounds. My heart would be racing out of my chest, and the girl that used to seek out social interactions just was not there anymore.

I found myself not wanting to answer the phone, and staying in, rather than associating with friends and family that I loved. It took me two hours to fall asleep at night, and then I would wake up multiple times in the night for no reason at all.

I chalked it up to having four kids in seven years, and being in my thirties. I had accepted that maybe I was becoming introverted, and FOR SURE young moms are just tired. Right??? Right???

I almost wore it like a badge of honor. I got through my days with sugar and naps. My entire world revolved around getting out of bed in the morning, hoping someone would show up with a binky and blanket for me to take a nap at 11:00am, which never happened. All the mamas with little ones KNOW!

I was happy, but in survival mode. As a positive person I have always been focused on the good, because life is too short to focus on the negative through hard times. I was worried though that if I did not change something, things would only get worse.

Who knew that something as simple as improving my gut health could transform EVERYTHING in my life? Not only is my extroverted self-back , but my racing heart, sugar cravings (plus the forty pounds of chocolate peanut butter ice cream that came with them), skin issues, hair falling out, sleep that never came, naps, and covers weighing 1,000 pounds in the morning are a thing of the past. A memory that I know was real, but feels more like a dream now. Not necessarily a bad one...just one that was so vividly part of my reality every day.

I love waking up alert for myself, my children, my friends, and my family. I share my story with you today so that if you or someone you know is silently suffering, you will know you are not alone and that there IS another way.

Who would have thought that gut health could do all of this?

Secret 2

The New Paradigm of Gut Health

Hippocrates said 'All disease begins in the gut.' We are finally coming full circle with the crystal clear message that he was right and now we need to get back to the root of the cause of disease and look at the gut to solve the problems. The 'New' paradigm is what we are now thinking is the new information that has really been here all along. Great philosophers knew it. We just strayed away from it.

Where along history did we get off track? I am not sure, but I am so glad we are circling back. It will become more apparent from learning about gut health that the health of your gut will impact your overall health both positively and negatively.

Gut Bacteria

90% of the cells in the gut are not human. They are microorganisms - bacteria and fungi that live in our gut and aid or detract from its function. The term microbiome used in this book refers to those microorganisms in our gut.

The term gut health is used in talking about the complete digestive system and all of the microorganisms, fungi and bacteria together and how they relate to each other and to the health of our bodies.

Gut bacteria that is in your microbiome protects against certain ailments. Some people may lack a good variety of bacteria or have too little or too many of specific types.

Gut bacteria affects your metabolism. It also affects how many calories you get from food and the nutrients that get absorbed from what you eat. Two people can eat the same meal and have different amounts of calories and nutrients absorbed into their bodies depending on the gut bacteria they each possess.

Have you ever noticed an overweight person who actually eats very little food each day yet he or she seems to stay the same size? Or a person who is very thin eats, and eats, and eats. You may think 'How can they eat so much and stay that size?' Each example should eventually have a dramatic change in the size or shape of his or her body if they kept eating very little or too much, yet the size of the person does not change the way you may think it should.

The study of gut health has come a long way. According to the World Health Organization's (WHO) definition of 'health' from 1948, 'health' is 'the absence of diseases.' One might also define 'gut health' as a state of physical and mental well-being in the absence of Gastro-intestinal (GI) complaints that require the consultation of a doctor. We now know gut health is so much more than that simple definition from 1948.

Gut health can offer a new approach to preventative medicine and that new approach to preventative medicine is how we can learn to achieve optimal health and maintain it.

Current medical research is much more focused on the treatment of defined GI diseases rather than on the prevention of disease. However, preventative medicine is increasing more and more, perceived to be as important in medical and economic terms.

The field of gastroenterology is a profession that has been studying more on the preventative approach to gut health. Gastroenterology scientifically justified approaches to gut health and to preventing GI diseases.

We have started to learn that lifestyle characteristics, such as eating a balanced diet, moderate but regular exercise, avoidance of chronic stress, and consistent use of supplements with prebiotics and probiotics can support gut health.

This topic will affect us even more in the future if we succeed at increasing our knowledge of gut health and how to influence it in a positive way.

Julia, a military wife from California started to exercise and make food changes, after developing health issues. These changes brought some relief, but when she began healing her gut she started seeing greater results. Healing her gut helped her reduce her medications and experience less flare ups in her body from inflammation.

I am jumping for joy because my rheumatologist said I had another round of great labs and is letting me wean down my anti-inflammatory injections again!!

About two years ago, I was diagnosed with an autoimmune condition called Psoriatic Arthritis. I had never heard of it before, but have seen several commercials since then talking about it and what medications are available to treat it.

It became the quiet thing that 'I had' just like people who 'have' insomnia, thyroid issues, crazy cravings, depression, anxiety, painful joints, allergies or asthma. Why are we so accepting of these and just treating the symptoms as they flare up vs. treating the root cause?

For me, for the first year I had this, I just did not know any other way. I did not understand the links between my symptoms and how daily balanced hormones and balancing my gut microbiome could heal me from those ailments.

My doctor said 'you will have this for the rest of your life.' I am so grateful I tried a different treatment, as skeptical as I was that it would work for me, and did not quit early on.

A year strong now and feeling the best I have in about a decade.

Four months ago after reading a book called The Adrenal Thyroid Revolution I dived into gut health research. From the outside I looked super healthy and happy, but inside I was struggling! I was averaging ten doctor visits a year.

I had struggled with postpartum depression following the birth of each of my children, thyroid issues, bloating and fatigue, symptoms of hypoglycemia, which were matched by sugar cravings since I was a kid.

I was diagnosed with my autoimmune condition a year ago, and I was injecting myself with anti-inflammatory medication weekly. I knew this was due to stress on my body. My youngest child suffered from febrile seizures and many of my own conditions appeared within just a few months of his first seizure.

I worked out and made food changes in my family, but my symptoms did not improve. After researching gut health, I started cutting out gluten for a month. I still craved sweets, still felt bloated, still had psoriasis. I decided to give some natural gut health supplements a try. I initially felt super skeptical, but also super hopeful that they would work.

Four and a half months in, and I have seen incredible changes. I went through digestive issues with Candida die off and did not notice much of a difference month's one and two. Month three was really my sweet spot where cravings really went down and I found myself passing on dessert nightly. I had not even thought to grab something sweet!

I sleep like a rock, I have more sustained energy and I have been able to stick to exercising three to four days a week (even going at 3 to 4pm in the afternoon - my previous dead time!). I have lost six lbs. - three of which were specifically from depression medications that I could not get off.

I do not get dizzy or weak if I am not constantly snacking. My depression and anxiety are a thing of the past... and to those of you that struggle with this, you will understand when I say that the lows come in life. The hardships do not disappear. What does fade is the length of time in the place you go to when they come. What used to last for days has faded much more quickly. It feels like a hard day, not an episode of depression.

Because I am more balanced, I am more resilient. More forgiving of others and myself.

A huge unexpected blessing came when I started opening my mouth about the changes I was seeing. We all talk about how teaching our kids service is the best way to stop focusing on yourself. When I started sharing what I had learned and started focusing on other people's health concerns, wanting them to find hope and success, there was less time to focus on my problems.

When I started getting comments on how for the first time in years someone was feeling relief, something changed within me. I wanted to help more and more people. I wanted others to feel alive again and to feel like the best versions of themselves.

Want to hear an even more incredible part? The best part of me, my kids, also had some health concerns. My eight year old had been dealing with anxiety and anger issues for about six to eight months and we were running out of home solutions. I started him on supplements in September. He had developed spring allergies and so far so good - no medications needed yet this year! Most importantly, his anxiety and anger issues have significantly decreased. We no longer worry about him and we have our sweet boy back.

My four year old the one with Febrile seizures, also has asthma. He had starting having seizures when he was one and a half. A few months into my routine, I put him on the same gut health supplements. He is supposed to grow out of the seizures and asthma by six, so I thought I would put these supplements to the test. We are now eight months into cold and flu season with zero visits to the doctor and emergency room.

No need for his inhalers. One short seizure, right before his dad left for Afghanistan, compared to the eight to ten per season each year prior. Since then we have had two short fevers with no accompanying seizures. I had canceled two gym memberships in the past once fall hit because I knew his immune system would get hit hard.

We had tried it all diet, exercise, less carbs, essential oils, and vitamins. I already changed my diet, exercised, I was eating less carbs and using essential oils, and it was not until I added in the RIGHT gut health supplements for me that I found the missing piece to the puzzle. I now continue to exercise and eat better while taking my supplements to have great gut health.

This year we are all here. Right now, together, really living.

Having a Healthy Gut

It is hard to know that you need to be educated in something you did not know existed. Well, now you know gut health exists! Now you know gut health is important. The question you may ask… how can you tell if you have a healthy gut?

A healthy gut consists of five main things. Number one is that you have effective digestion and absorption of food. Number two is an absence of Gastrointestinal (GI) illness. Number three is that you have a normal and stable intestinal microbiome. Number four is an effective immune status. And number five is a status of well-being. Now let's talk about each of these a little more.

Number One- Effective digestion and absorption of food means having your nutritional needs met, having the proper absorption of food, water and minerals. Effective digestion is also having regular bowel movements with normal transit time and without abdominal pain. Regular bowel movements is having one to two bowels movements each day (yes, we will be talking about poop a lot in this book, and going to the bathroom once a week is not normal). It is best to eat three times a day and poop three times a day. You should have a normal stool consistency (light brown and floats), without nausea, vomiting, diarrhea, constipation or bloating.

Number Two- Absence of GI illness means no acid peptic disease, reflux disease or other gastric inflammatory disease; no enzyme deficiencies or carbohydrate intolerances, no inflammatory bowel diseases (IBD), colon disease or other inflammatory state, and no colon or other GI cancer.

Number Three- Normal and balanced intestinal microbiome means no bacterial or yeast overgrowth and a happy and healthy gut microbiome, no GI infections or antibiotic-associated diarrhea. Candida (yeast) overgrowth is a big problem for many people and most people do not even know it exists, let alone that it is a contributing factor in their health issues. Candida is needed in the body in small amounts and controlled; it is when it has an overgrowth that it can cause health issues in the body.

Number Four- Effective immune status means having an effective GI barrier function, normal mucus production and no enhanced bacterial translocation. The term 'bacterial translocation' is used to describe the passage of bacteria from the gastrointestinal tract to tissues such as the lymph nodes and other internal organs. Translocation is the movement of something from one place to another, so in terms you can understand bacteria gets passed from the intestines to healthy organs. An effective immune status also includes normal levels of IgA (immunoglobulin A), normal numbers (a doctor can help you know what is normal for you), and normal activity of immune cells. It also includes immune tolerance and no allergy or mucous hypersensitivity.

Number Five- Status of well-being means a normal quality of life, a healthy mental state, positive gut feeling, balanced serotonin production, and normal function of the entire nervous system.

After improving her gut health Jessica C. decided to take that knowledge and make a career with it. That career involves helping others learn about gut health and what products they can take to improve their health naturally.

Hey Guys, My name is Jessica C. My husband and I raise our four wildly, adorable boys in a tiny, little town in Southeast Idaho.

Twenty-one months ago I was not in a good place. Health wise things were a mess. I had a number of health conditions that started very early in my life. I have had an Inflammatory Bowel Disease for the last twenty years, which also affected my immune system, because of this I had chronic infections.

As you can imagine both of these health issues left me feeling pretty miserable. I had to stay close to a bathroom at all times, and so I missed out on a lot of family activities. I was always exhausted and my kids had to literally pull me out of bed. Anytime my kids needed me, they came looking in my bed or in the bathroom. I lived on caffeinated soda, energy drinks and tea. I woke up most mornings with headaches. I was moody and irritable. This was no fun for anyone.

I have been on gut health supplements for a little over twenty-one months now, and my health still has its challenges, but is night and day better!!!

Not being able to work outside of the home, left us swimming in debt. When a new bill came in, I just laughed at it, made an airplane out of it, or shook my head at it and repeated, 'That Poor Secretary!!!' She just wasted her time sending me this bill... because it ain't getting paid. Sometimes I used to think, maybe they would rather have monopoly money, then a check that would most often bounce.

Life was rough!!! You know how people say, they 'Live paycheck to paycheck???' Well for almost thirteen years we have lived paycheck to five minutes later after it would hit the bank. Over the years, I became an amazing couponer. A pro at searching through racks at the second hand stores, I was pretty dang good at finding a deal on everything. I had to be. When we would go out as a family for a treat, I played a game called, 'Will it or won't it' It was always nerve racking waiting for the waitress to declare if the transaction was approved or declined.

No matter how hard my husband worked, (and trust me, he works his fanny off!!!) We could never get ahead. Each month we got further and further in the hole. Why....Do I tell you all this??? Because twenty-one months ago I prayed for supplements to be the miracle that my health desperately needed. What I did not expect was for it to be the miracle that my finances needed.

As I started sharing with my friends and family, who I knew needed gut health products, I never imagined I would start creating an income. We ain't talkin 'HOBBY' money, but 'PAY YO BILLS' kind of money. I had never been rewarded for sharing something that I loved, in such a way. No restaurant or clothing line had ever sent me a check, for recommending something that I Loved, but my supplement line of products does.

After the first few weeks, I paid for my products. First Month, I paid for a plane ticket to be with my mother who was having emergency surgery. I remember being so proud, and blessed that I could be with her.

About month four to five I was able to make my car payment and other misc bills. Month six paid for a month of groceries for a house of six (five being boys). After.... Twenty-one months, I have made my mortgage and new car payment. And just last month we bought a new four-wheeler and dirt bikes for the boys. 'Merry Christmas and Happy Birthday!!!!!!'

Last week (month twenty-one) we just found out daddy was laid off for the next several months. AM I freaking out!?!?! Not gonna Lie... I am a little, but the truth is, last time this happened he was 100% of our income. Now I make half as much as he does, so guess what that means??? Our needs are going to be covered, and all will be OK. You can't imagine the stress that I am relieving from him, from myself!

We have been truly blessed by these gut health supplements, in sooo many ways, but these are my favorites.

*My entire family uses these products and have better health
*I can put all my kids in sports, and music
*Shipping diapers to a family member who struggles
*Treating friends to the movie theater who never go
*Surprising a family with Christmas
*Making bags to hand out to the homeless
*Family vacations/family time

These might seem like little things but these are some of the things that I can do now because of learning about great natural gut health supplements. Because I share with family and friends. Because I share something that will help them live a happier and healthier life.

I love that with this great line of gut health supplements I can choose to work full time or part time, and I get to do it with babies on my lap.

Dysbiosis

Are you still not convinced of the importance of improving your gut health? Here is another reason why it is important for you to care. There is a massive amount of bacteria inside you. Most of which is not human, which is kind of gross to think about, but there are ten times as many bacteria in your body than there are human cells. Furthermore, there is one hundred times the amount of bacteria DNA in your body than human DNA. So you could argue that you are more bacterial than you are human.

Before you start to freak out, the majority of the bacteria in your microbiome are vitally important for digesting food, developing your immune system, and protecting you from harmful bacteria.

Your gut bacteria are constantly telling your immune system what to do. Did you know that bacteria can send signals to the intestines and back again? This communication can cause your immune system to make adjustments to regulations of your body and how it will respond when needed. Your gut is a second brain for your body, called the Gut-Brain connection (we will talk more about this a little later).

Your microbiome is constantly changing. Do you want to be in charge of these changes or just leave it up to chance? When you are not paying attention to your health you are running the risk of that microbiome changing negatively instead of positively. These changes help your body learn what needs to be done and how to react. The body is constantly absorbing food, bacteria, viruses, fungi, and parasites from the outside world. The gathering of these microbes and particles is basically an accumulation of all your most recent bodily experiences.

Just like a daily journal of your adventures, your body keeps track of all the different comings and goings of bacteria. When bacteria particles come in contact with the inner lining of your intestines, which is packed full of immune cells, the cells constantly sample all of the particles that it comes into contact with. When new bacteria venture in, the body has to separate good bacteria and bad bacteria. The body then decides, whether to play nice or attack and protect.

Your microbiome needs to maintain balance and when that balance is disrupted dysbiosis occurs. Dysbiosis can seriously affect the scale of your health.

Depending on the severity of dysbiosis in the gut exposure to certain conditions can negatively affect one person while having minimal change to another person.

Have you ever traveled and tried a new restaurant only to get sick the next day? Have you finished a high stress project at work, only to get sick right afterward? Have you eaten a frozen burrito for lunch when you normally eat a salad, and then felt sick and bloated? Your body should have the ability to return to its 'normal' microbiome after being exposed to the conditions of change, but sometimes it cannot. This becomes a concern and the effects become more imbalanced with the new changes. This imbalance is what causes dysbiosis.

Even though professional researchers are constantly learning new things, it is increasingly more apparent that there is so much more we do not know. There is one thing that is certain; you should take care of your little microbial buddies as much as possible. After feeding your microbiome buddies a great diet, probiotics, and supplements, they will start to thrive and you will see positive changes happening in your gut and in your body.

Secret 3

Your Microbiome, Everybody's Got One

The microbiome has been referred to as our 'forgotten organ.' Just like a fingerprint, each person's microbiome is unique. Your microbiome is determined partly from your mother's microbiome that you were exposed to at birth and partly from your lifestyle, diet, and environment you live in.

Your microbiome starts to develop in the early stages of life, starting when babies passing through the birth canal become coated with microbes from their mothers. Then the infants are exposed to a variety of other bacteria encountered in breast milk and the environment. This helps the microbiome grow and become customized by the time the child is 3 years old. The first few years of a child's life is critical in how that microbiome is developed. What happens in the developing of the microbiome in these years can be factors that determine diseases and symptoms that develop later in life. As babies begin to eat more complex foods, microbes assist by releasing enzymes to help in the digestion of nutrients. As we get older the bacteria in our gut affects us more and more. It grows and becomes more complex in supporting functions of the body like aiding in the active digestive juices, and producing vitamins including vitamin K.

Research also shows that our gut bacteria can also alter how our bodies store fat, balance glucose levels in the blood, and respond to hormones that make us feel hungry. The microbiome develops alongside our immune system.

This complex network of cells, tissues, and organs defend and support the body against invading viruses and bacteria that cause disease and inflammation. Eighty percent of the immune system is located in the gut. Here beneficial microbes form a line of defense against the attack of germs and viruses. Studies show that some of those microbes can even release their own antibiotics to fight invaders.

You can change your microbiome; just because you are born with it does not mean you have to stick to it. What you have now is not set in stone, through health adjustments and environment adjustments you can slowly alter you microbiome for the better or worse.

Of the thousands of species of bacteria in the microbiome (which can be over three pounds) each plays a different role in your body. These bacteria contain over two million genes. Most of the bacteria are extremely important for your health, while some can cause disease. The microbes in your intestines, act as another organ that is crucial for your health.

The gut microbiome affects the body from birth and throughout life by controlling digestion of food, immune and central nervous systems, heart, weight, and many other bodily processes and aspects of health. Your body is one thing you have to take care of from birth until death. You only get one body; there is no trading it in.

Dani, mom of two little ones realized that gut health does not always have to do with the scale. Dani shares how child birth is something that had a drastic effect on her microbiome.

I felt prompted to share some of my many non-scale related gut health victories with you all today. And one is very near and dear to my heart.

My first daughter and I always had a very up and down nursing relationship. I always had the idea that I wanted to nurse her and give her breast milk for the first year of her life. Nothing against formula feeding, this was just my personal goal. Well, at three months my baby decided to stop taking a bottle. So it was all mom, all the time.

What made this more challenging was that from the very beginning, I started getting clogged ducts and milk blisters. Do you know what a milk blister is? If yes, I need to say no more. If not, be grateful. I would get them multiple times a month and the pain would sometimes last a week. I even had multiple ones at the same time. Not to go into too much detail, they got so bad that it was affecting my baby.

I was told to change my diet, eliminate dairy, nuts, some meats, chocolate, spinach, and some other things... um... yeah no. I took two to three lecithin tablets a day hoping it would help. It never really did but I was determined to keep providing for my baby for her first year.

Then I added in natural gut health supplements to my routine. The thought crossed my mind that these may help, but it was not something I was expecting. Guess what? Not. One. Single. Problem. NONE. Nothing from the very beginning!! No clogged ducts, milk blebs (blister), or engorgement (sorry boys). I cannot tell you how grateful I was to finally have a good nursing relationship with my little one!!

I also went from having migraines and chronic back aches to being able to haul my baby around and hitting up the gym for workouts. I walk and jog with the jogging stroller multiple times a week. I love watching these supplements change lives, especially when it is my family? Who in your family needs to heal their gut?

I carried around an inhaler everywhere I went for about five years. When I first noticed breathing problems, it felt like there was a huge pressure on my chest and I had to concentrate on deeply breathing in and out or else I did not feel like I was getting any air, so my doctor prescribed a little breathing helper. I usually took it once a day at most, sometimes less, sometimes more. Always before or after working out. During certain times of the year it would get worse depending on where we were living at the time. I hated taking it. Sometimes it made me feel light headed, and once in a while I could feel my heart beating differently.

Well, the other day my husband asked, 'when was the last time I needed that inhaler?' Hhmm... good question, I said. I cannot remember! So I thought back. And... I had used it ONCE in the last year since starting my supplements. Say what?! And the other morning during my jog/walk workout I could BREATHE fully and deeply with no help needed and I had to smile and send a little prayer of thanks.

No longer do I need to be inconvenienced by this little device. No longer do I need to worry that I could get a breathing attack when I was just playing with my kids. No longer do I need to worry about the short and long term effects of continued use.

I can tell you that getting my gut healthy and reducing inflammation in my body has gotten to the root issue of my breathing problems. And I do not need medicine with side effects!

Now after baby number two, I am still enjoying my gut health products.

When my first baby was little, a baby carrier was a no-go for me. It did not matter how I wore her, it would always hurt my lower back. Good thing she did not like it much anyway. Now with my second, I find myself being able to wear my baby whenever I want. One day a few months ago I even realized I had been wearing her for four hours straight! I was amazed and my back felt fine.

I am so grateful that I do not have to worry about how I am going to do something or go somewhere where a stroller might not go, or where my baby would not sit still for long enough. I have got my carrier and I am good to go!

What changed? I got to the root of my pain issues - inflammation. Am I always pain free? Nope. Because I do not live a perfect life. Sometimes I eat something that flares up that inflammation and I can feel it. But not the way I used to. It is a lot less and a lot more manageable.

Who knew the right kind of gut health supplements could heal so many issues I have had over the years?

Your Gut Garden

Think of your gut microbiome like a garden. Picture in your mind a large beautiful garden. Your garden should be a garden full of a large variety of healthy plants; it should be continually growing and flourishing. All the different species of good gut flora, bacteria, fungi and even viruses are the variety of plants growing in your garden. In your garden should be a large variety of wonderful and useful plants. These plants 'do good' in the body and keep everything functioning the way God created it to function.

There may be a few weeds (bad bacteria, fungi, yeast, or viruses) popping up every now and then, but when you have a happy, healthy garden, the weeds will not thrive because the immune system in the body can attack those weeds and keep them under control.

When something like an antibiotic is taken into the body, it wipes out the entire garden of both the good and the bad plants. It is like pouring weed killer on your garden, and it destroys everything. When you have a large, barren area of soil, what tends to flourish? The weeds!

The weeds grow much faster than the good plants. They can grow with little nourishment or water. So now instead of a healthy garden, you have a garden where the good flora (plants) has little chance of survival. The weeds overpower any little seeds trying to peek through. The good plants do not stand a chance.

Now you will want to plant some seeds (probiotics for new good bacteria) back in your garden and repopulate the good plants. If every spring you planted seeds in a garden full of weeds, how well do you think those seeds would grow? They may even be high quality seeds and you may be taking good care to feed them, but they will still have a hard time thriving unless you are weeding at the same time. You need to constantly weed your garden so the new seeds can grow.

Now you have weeded and you have planted your new seeds, do you just walk away and hope that they flourish? Do you think that new weeds will never pop back up and try to crowd out the good again? Taking care of the garden is a constant job, one that needs to be tended to on a daily basis.

With proper love and care the garden can be like it once was, happy, healthy and flourishing. That garden can protect the body from weed attacks. That garden can build up the immune system so it can work at maximum capacity. Does it mean the body will never get sick? No, but does it mean that the body will have its best, and strongest line of defense ready for war, Yes!

Just like the body needs food and water every day to survive, the microbiome needs constant nourishment to keep the garden growing well. So, what happens when we never tend to the garden and the weeds overrun? Those weeds grow strong roots, and those roots spread out all over the microbiome, throughout the gut, and other parts of the body. These roots have many names; one well-known name of yeast is Candida.

Candida

Candida yeast, which is a form of fungus, lives in your mouth and intestines in very small amounts. Candida aids in digestion and nutrient absorption. When this yeast is overproduced in the body it can cause an overgrowth of yeast or Candida overgrowth. When talking about this overgrowth of yeast the term Candida may be used by itself but will be referring to a Candida overgrowth in the body.

When there is an overgrowth of Candida this overgrowth breaks down the wall of the intestine and penetrates the bloodstream. Candida then spreads through the body causing havoc. It attacks the body's immune system, it creates inflammation, it can even cause mystery illness and symptoms where no one knows what is wrong, just pain and discomfort.

Candida feeds on sugar, carbohydrates, medication, birth control, stress, and poor diet choices. It grows fast and out of control. Think about what happens when you add sugar to warm yeast when cooking or baking. It expands rapidly. It also is very hard to attack. It has a hard shell that has to be broken down to be eliminated. Diet and exercise can help greatly but sometimes supplements, probiotics, and enzymes need to be used to attack it and bring it back into a controlled amount.

Candida can invade every tissue in the body as well as the brain. Candida grows and thrives on what you eat and makes your body crave what it needs to survive. This is the reason Candida can be difficult to eradicate from the body, but it can be controlled with proper steps.

Candida can be present alongside many health issues. Interestingly, about 80% of fibromyalgia sufferers also have Candida. This may be the case with many health issues. Candida is there and you do not even know it.

Candida can occasionally occur alone, but more often than not, it is related to other health issues.

Take for example the symptoms of Candida and fibromyalgia. Symptoms are the same, with the exception of hot spots or touch points common to fibromyalgia sufferers. Both Candida and fibromyalgia are auto-immune disorders. Someone with both conditions should address and treat Candida while addressing the fibromyalgia.

Candida can lie dormant for up to six months. When your heath is back in control, keep in mind that Candida is always ready and able to spring back into life if it is fed. Even after you heal the gut you have to keep the Candida in balance. It is not something that you fix and it stays put, it is ever changing. You can help to keep it in balance with a proper diet, exercise and supplementation.

Microbiome Testing

There are ways to harness the power of your microbiome and as we continue to gain a greater knowledge of that power and what it can do, there are companies already appealing to the health conscious consumers.

Microbiome testing at home is a way you can evaluate your gut health. It is very simple to do. You purchase a test and send in a stool sample (yes you send your poop in the mail), mouth swab, vaginal swab or other requirements. The company will then send you results with recommendations or evaluations as to how you rate compared to others.

Depending on the company they might make food, diet, or other recommendations to help improve your microbiome to increase your overall gut health. Some companies have an at-home kit delivered once a year, with options to repeat the test whenever you desire. Other companies have an artificial intelligence engine trained by leading gut scientists, physicians, and nutritionists that analyze and prepare a personalized, easy-to-follow plan with diet, nutrition and supplement recommendations delivered via a proprietary app.

There are more and more companies sprouting up with these great services so people can take control of their health and learn more as to how to improve their own health.

Kimberly, mom of five from Colorado, knows how important test results can be in understanding the health of the gut. Kimberly explains,

I want to share my gut health reality. I am so emotional from my quick results. After adding in gut health supplements the results are changing my life. I feel amazing!

My body is healing inside and out! Better digestion, no headaches, better skin, almost no back aches, no cravings for carbohydrates, more energy, more mental clarity, the list keeps going! I am working out every day and I have cut my carbohydrates down, but my cravings are no longer there, so this helps! I no longer have severe depression and hypothyroidism and I am off my anxiety medications.

I love that I am now present in my kid's life. I look forward to days of playing with them, hiking, riding scooters, and enjoying life. It feels so good to feel good!

My dad also shared with me that he had his semi-annual health check after incorporating gut health supplements. His doctor was ecstatic A1C dropped almost a full point. His LDL dropped 76 points to 55. His HDL is up, Blood pressure after coming from work was 110/61 and he has lost 27 lbs.

His doctor said his next visit he will start taking him off some meds! Blood pressure, blood sugar, and cholesterol meds, all to be reduced. The best thing he has ever done was start on gut health supplements. When you follow the regimen good things happen!!!

Are your parents on supplements? Are they on medication? I encourage you to get them started on healing their gut. I know it has been a huge change for me and my family!

Secret 4

Signs That Your Gut is Out of Whack

Symptoms of poor gut health can be a variety of things, which can also be signs or symptoms of other health issues. If you have any of these symptoms you will need to check with a doctor to see if they are related to poor gut health or if you may have other health issues that are causing these symptoms.

Irritable bowel syndrome (IBS), compromise flatulence, bloating, regurgitation, heartburn, nausea, vomiting, constipation, diarrhea, food intolerance, abnormal pain and cramps, loss of appetite, allergies, mood or mental health issues, skin issues, weight gain, brain fog, lack of concentration, and thyroid issues are all symptoms related to poor gut health.

More symptoms can also include anorexia, unintended weight loss, dysphagia (difficulty swallowing), continued vomiting, severe abdominal pain or diarrhea, melena (upper gastrointestinal bleeding) and hematochezia (blood in stools).

Gut health is coming up more and more in medical conversations and how important it is, but it is rarely tested. There is so much written about it but many people are still uneducated because the way it is defined and what constitutes wellness and a healthy gut are not clear.

Diagnosing poor gut health is hard to do because there is no real baseline to start with.

Julie is a Sergeant with the State Police. She is forty years old and a mother of three. She grew up in a small town. She was the second of five kids and grew up on a ranch with both sets of grandparents next door. Julie struggled for years with health issues until she realized it was all related to her gut being out of whack from traumatic events in her life. Julie shares

I was your typical tomboy and loved to be outside.

My dad had a ranch, an excavation business, a mechanic shop, and he did pretty much anything and everything to pay the bills. I was his right hand man and even though it was hard work I enjoyed getting dirty every day.

I really enjoy operating heavy equipment and driving a truck. I went to school in a kindergarten through twelfth grade schoolhouse. I graduated with eight in my class. I was hired by the State Police in 2002 and soon after that my dad was diagnosed with Parkinson's disease. It was devastating for him. It was progressing rapidly.

My husband is also a Sergeant for the State Police. He started a couple years after I did and says that he knew he wanted to marry me before he even met me.

I was promoted to detective in 2005 and started to gain weight. I was not eating very good and spent the majority of my time at work sitting in my car or sitting at the office. We got married in 2006, and we started trying to get pregnant right away but then I was diagnosed with PCOS (Polycystic Ovary Syndrome).

I had never had a regular cycle. My cycle is extremely heavy and comes whenever it wants. I had to use super plus tampons and an overnight pad that I would change every couple hours. This would last ten days or more. I had such bad cramps that all I wanted to do is curl up on the couch with a hot pad. I had terrible migraines and would feel weak during this time. I was put on fertility drugs which are miserable. I gave up with fertility stuff and we then had our first child in 2008.

Pregnancy was extremely hard on me. I had morning sickness for the entire nine months. I actually lost weight during pregnancy and herniated a disc in my back shortly after giving birth to a beautiful baby girl. During maternity leave I would use the stroller in the house to transport my baby because I could barely walk. I quickly gained the weight back and more. I saw lots of doctors for my back pain and was told surgery was my only option. I was too stubborn for that. I tried anti-inflammatory shots, pain pills, and a chiropractor. Nothing seemed to work. After returning to work, I quickly lost my milk supply and was not able to nurse. I wanted to nurse and this caused me to resent myself.

In 2010, I had my second child, a son. I did not have morning sickness quite as bad, but it lasted almost 9 months. I again lost weight during pregnancy and herniated another disc after delivery. Now I had one running around and another to care for. My husband did not take very much time off work, but he helped on his days off. I had to go on antidepressants and the longer I took them the more I hated myself for having to take them. My husband wanted to have more children and even though I knew pregnancy was not fun I wanted him to be happy.

During late 2012, I got pregnant with my second daughter. In February 2013, I had a bleeding episode and was taken to the hospital by ambulance. Work was extremely stressful and I lacked the ability to cope. On top of that an individual I worked with and I were not getting along. I was extremely emotional and did not handle things appropriately. I also suffered period back pain that was so severe that I could not walk.

My son was a mamma's boy and busy busy. In May 2013, I had a severe gall bladder attack that sent me into labor and I was life-flighted to the hospital. I was put on bed-

rest and had a beautiful baby girl in July. She did not cry and needed special attention.

The doctors and nurses had left me alone in my room for 2 hours right after delivery. I had an epidural and I could not get my legs to work. I finally got them to work enough to get out of bed and go to the bathroom. They were still numb but I made my way to the nursery to find my baby. I was shocked when I realized they had her on a high dose of oxygen.

I tried to nurse her, but she would not eat. I am a very over protective momma and it was really stressful not having my baby with me at all times. That night they woke me up at 2 a.m. They told me that she had an apneic episode and they wanted to do a spinal tap. When I walked into the room the doctor was telling the nurse that the needle was too big and wanted a smaller one. The nurses stated that they did not have one and when the doctor said OK I will try this one, I stopped him and said 'no you won't.' You will ship us somewhere that has the correct needle.

They sent us to another hospital where one doctor thought she was having seizures. They ran all sorts of tests and the specialist did not think she was having seizures. Most of the episodes occurred when I had stepped away to either sleep or eat. The tests showed nothing other than abnormal brain activity.

We spent a few weeks at the hospital before the doctor decided that he could not do anything and sent us to a Children's Hospital. One life-flight costs $250,000. This was our second flight in one year. I cannot even remember how much per day the NICU cost, but I worried every day how I was going to pay the bills.

With this high stress in my life I was not taking care of myself. I had terribly high blood pressure and swollen legs. As you can imagine I was not eating right and I got terrible mastitis from not pumping effectively. While at the Children's

Hospital they decided to move her feeding tube and perforated her bowel. My sweet little angel never recovered. In August 2013, she died. After the funeral I had gall bladder removal surgery and as soon as I recovered from that I returned to work.

In February 2014, I was promoted to detective Sergeant and moved for the job. The move was a mess. I could not pack because of my back pain and the rental was not ready for us to move in. It was filthy. The carpet was coming apart and there was blood on the bathroom door. It was just nasty.

I was not welcomed with open arms. The guys in the office were very upset that I got the job over the other detective that applied and immediately started causing problems for me. They were recording me and trying to get me in trouble. My boss was gone for most of the first year. I had my car broken into and my gun stolen. I was extremely overweight. I also was suffering from severe allergies and vertigo episodes. The house we were living in had the carpet replaced and new paint, but I was still so sick.

The patrol lieutenant was encouraging the guys to record me and when I brought it to the Captain's attention I was told that he was not doing anything wrong. In the fall I was put on administrative leave and accused of lying by my boss, the detective lieutenant. I was put on what I call house arrest. During the weekdays I could not leave my house between the hours of 8 am and 5 pm. I sat for months in my house wondering what was going on at work, thinking that I needed to be there, and trying to figure out what I did wrong. I luckily was skeptical of a meeting I had with my captain and lieutenant and recorded that meeting myself.

That recording saved my job. The captain was asked to retire and the lieutenant was given days off. Now I had to work for this lieutenant knowing that he lied and that he did not get the same house arrest treatment that I got. He did not even have to tell the detectives in the office that he got in trouble for accusing me of lying. He just told them that he took some vacation.

A few months later I was sexually harassed and I made the mistake of letting my lieutenant know. He put the detective on administrative leave before I could handle it myself. This did not help me build a relationship with the detectives. The lieutenant did other things that caused me problems and I was told that I needed to work it out with him. The detective came back from administrative leave and I was told that a subordinate cannot sexually harass a boss and I should have done something about it as his supervisor.

I had worked hard to earn my job with the State Police and I was not giving it up. I love the agency and I had quit too many other things in the past. During this time I had to have my tonsils removed which is not fun for an adult and my health was depleting.

I finished two years as a detective sergeant and transferred to patrol sergeant. Now I worked for the lying patrol lieutenant that encouraged the detectives to record me. I was not happy to go to work every day. I had been out of patrol for eleven years. A lot had changed and I had not received any training. I did not know how to operate the radio or the computer programs. When I left patrol, years before, we did not have computers in the cars and we had VHS recording systems. Now my camera records to an SD card and everything is computerized. I not only had to learn how to patrol again, but I had to supervise a team. I had a young team and I seized the opportunity for a fresh start. I wanted to be a great Sergeant.

On my days off I would literally veg out the entire day. As soon as I got home I would take off my uniform and sit down. I was so tired I barely had enough energy to feed my kids and keep them alive. I still had severe depression, but I was not taking the medicine anymore. My cycles were more painful and heavier than they had ever been. I had terrible migraines and my allergies were out of control. I was sick so often and every cold turned into a sinus infection. I was taking antibiotics every couple of months. I did not cope very well with the loss of my daughter and blamed myself. I had terrible nightmares and I would 'what if' every chance I got.

I have suffered my entire life with IBS and anxiety. I have never slept very well and any little bit of stress would keep me awake. I could not attend a house party without feeling claustrophobic. A group of more than 2-3 people was too much for me to handle. Anytime I ate I had to run to the bathroom. It is not very convenient while in uniform to go to the bathroom, so I would not eat, yet I continued to gain weight.

I segregated myself from everyone. I un-friended friends and felt so betrayed by God, and my friends while I was going through these trials. I was snappy with my kids and impatient with them. I would cry uncontrollably sometimes and I craved salty fast food. I had made the decision to take the promotion and I felt it was my fault. I grew that baby girl in my belly for 9 months and I felt responsible that I had caused all her problems.

In March 2017, I was introduced to some gut health supplements that changed my life. Within a few days I felt like going for a walk with my daughter and I was not as tired. Then I felt like running. I also started sleeping better. I work 'shift work' and it did not matter when I got to bed I would fall asleep within a short period of time. Within a few weeks I was actually constipated which was a new thing for me.

Over the last year I have only had one vertigo episode. My IBS is gone. My anxiety is controllable and I have started making friends. Stores do not stress me out anymore and I do not find myself running to the bathroom. I sleep like a teenager *and I only have had one cold (I ran out of my probiotic for a couple weeks and I caught a severe cold), but no sinus infections. My back is unbelievably better. I can run, exercise, and still be able to walk the next day. I have lost a little bit of weight, but mostly inches. I crave water instead of fast food. I have more mental clarity and a lot more patience. My cycles come every month on time, only last for 3 days, and are light and symptom free. I have been able to complete our fitness test and still be able to walk the next day. I have never been happier.*

I have researched how trauma affects gut health and I would say that I have had trauma in my life. Some days I want to slap my forehead and say 'duh,' how did I not think about gut health as being an answer sooner? The best part about getting my gut under control is that I am now enjoying my kids. They are so busy and so much fun.

My dad is also seeing benefits from improving his gut health. He has been able to reduce his Parkinson's medication, which is unheard of. Normally you slowly increase the dose until the medicine quits working and then you move to a stronger medicine. Because he is able to reduce the dose of the medicine it will work longer.

He is regular. He has fought constipation his entire life and needed help to eliminate. He is not consistent with his supplements and so the benefits come and go. I think that is where I got my stubborn side.

He does not seem to be as depressed or nearly as anxious. He is able to go out in public and not feel self-conscious about his shaking. He used to be a homebody and not want to go anywhere. He has been traveling more with my mom and they even went on vacation to the Oregon coast. His blood pressure and cholesterol are down. His doctor has approved his gut health supplements and told him to keep taking what he is taking.

Your Gut Health History

We are continually learning more and more about gut health and what causes damage to it. Evaluating someone's health history as it pertains to gut health includes a person's life history, including birth and childhood. The history has to include environment, stress, prescriptions, birth control, and other medications, diet, eating habits, life events, and exercise all discussed with a doctor.

A doctor can perform tests and analyze the results with all the factors that take place to evaluate the health of a person's gut. Such an approach requires the doctor to have validated tools for bowel-related complaints and symptoms that would enable doctors and clinics to record improvements in well-being, the quality of life and prognosis in selected populations.

Other environmental factors can contribute to the health of our microbiome that we do not even think about. How about obsessions with being clean? Cleanliness might actually be harming you. That does not mean I want everyone to start being dirty all the time and never clean up, but cleaners can be overused and be harmful. They are a great creation but sanitary wipes and anti-bacteria sanitizers that are marked as products to help us prevent illness and the spreading of germs are not that healthy for us.

Some sanitizers contain Triclosan which only targets certain types of bacteria. The creation of these products has even contributed to the creation of superbugs. Superbugs are a strain of bacteria that have become resistant to antibiotic drugs. If soap and water, which is best to use, are not around then make sure you are using an alcohol based hand sanitizer for your germs.

The lack of going outdoors can also be contributing to the health of your gut. People do not open windows or go outside as much. Exposure to a broad range of environments, including the ones outside in nature can actually improve microbial diversity in the gut. Americans spend only an estimate 5% of time outdoors. So open a window, open a door, take off your shoes and go for a walk outside.

Most of the time people spend outside is also spent on artificial ground. Enjoy nature, get outside, put your bare feet on the grass, dirt, anything to help ground your spirits and be exposed to a little bit of environmental bacteria. We need to interact with our earth. Exposure to the earth helps to stimulate our immune system over time.

Have you ever walked along the beach or on the grass in a park and just had that peaceful feeling about you? The Earth is an electrical planet, and you are a bio-electrical being living on an electrical planet. Your body functions electrically. Your heart and nervous system are prime examples. The earth below your feet provide what is compared as an electrical nutrition for your body.

Go barefoot for forty minutes outside and see what a difference that makes on your pain or stress level. Sit, stand, or walk on grass, sand, dirt, or concrete – preferably wet, for greater conduction of the Earth's electrons. These are all conductive surfaces from which your body can draw the Earth's electrons. Wood, asphalt, and vinyl are not conductive. Think of the soles of your shoes, what they are made of, if it is a man-made product, you may want to take them off to get a better conductive surface for your feet.

Other simple ways to realize your gut is out of whack is to answer these simple statements. Do you catch every bug that goes around? Do you or family members always seem to get sick and continually pass it back and forth when you get sick? Eighty percent of your immune system resides in your gut. If you are constantly sick then your gut is not balanced.

Do you have an itchy, blistery rash on your elbows and knees? It may look like eczema, but it could be Celiac disease, an autoimmune condition that makes you super sensitive to gluten. Many people go around for years being misdiagnosed only to end up with a worse condition because they let it go for so long untreated.

Do your teeth not look as white as they used to be? If your dentist has mentioned that the enamel on your teeth is worn down, you may want to go see a GI specialist. This can be a sign of undiagnosed Gastro Esophageal Reflux Disease (GERD), or acid reflux. Having a subtle sore throat, wheezing, and/or coughing can be a symptom as well. When sugary foods erode enamel, the front teeth are the ones that usually get damaged.

Are you depressed? Comfort foods may make you feel better temporarily, but they may be making your mood even worse. Fifty percent of dopamine and 90% of your serotonin is produced in the gut and when those poor food choices, or other contributing factors feed the bad bacteria it can cause symptoms of depression and anxiety to appear, or worsen.

Are you achy or feel wiped out all the time? When your bad bacteria get abnormally high in unbalanced levels it can appear in symptoms as vague as body aches, fatigue, and even diarrhea. The bad bacteria can interfere with your body's ability to break down and digest food and trigger vitamin and mineral deficiencies that zap all the energy from your body.

These are just a few simple ways to evaluate your gut. There are many more signs and symptoms to dive deeper into and see if you need to take a closer look at your gut. Share with your doctor if you have concerns with signs or symptoms when evaluating the health of your gut.

54

Secret 5

Gut-Brain Connection: Get Smart

What is the Gut-Brain Connection?

Our bodies and brains have always worked together, one affecting the other. Modern science has become aware of the fact that the brain effects the body, but they are just starting to understand how the body can affect the brain. This is how the gut and the brain are connected both ways not just as a one way direction.

Claire, foot zoner and board member of the Utah Foot Zone Association is well educated in the Gut-Brain connection and shares how a client changed her life for good.

I am a foot zoner and to promote my business I gave a couple of foot zoning sessions to be used at a raffle. A new client won the raffle. When she walked in my door, my life changed. I had been battling gut health for some time.

I have had multiple ulcer events. I have been scoped regularly. But even more important my body was not releasing the waste on a regular basis. With all of this in play, I had ballooned to 300lbs. This is not a cool thing when you are trying to help people with health.

As I zoned my new client, it became clear that she was one of the healthiest people I had worked on. I finally stopped and said, 'Why, are you here?' She told me she had come for a confirmation and told me how her life had changed because she had taken care of her gut.

I started on that same road and 50 lbs. later, (recognizing that I still have more to lose) I feel like I have reclaimed my life. In saying that, I want to make it perfectly clear that I did it through a system of gut health supplements and diet. It takes both. For me, I gave up dairy, soy and gluten. I also did not eat after 5 p.m. You have to have a plan in place to be successful.

The energy that came and the body confidence that was achieved was invaluable. Gut health, I now believe is at the center of everything.

Your Second Brain

All physical responses in our body have an emotional response as well. If you tell your body something long enough it will start to believe it to be true. Have you ever heard of positive talk? It is true how it can affect you for the good and the bad. We need to remember this as we discuss our gut health. How are we treating our bodies and what are we saying to ourselves have a direct relation to our gut health?

What are we saying verbally and nonverbally as we take care of our bodies and what we think of our self is reflected in our self-image? This also applies to our spirits. We need to know our spirit and our mind are connected and they listen to every hurtful thing we say to our self, even if it is unconscious.

Scientists refer to the gut as our second brain. This idea has been reflected in such great books like *The Good Gut, Brainmaker, The Microbiome Solution, and The Gut Balance Revolution.*

So test out some positive talk and start saying it to yourself every day. Come up with a positive affirmation or a mission statement. Repeat it several times morning and night. Your mind will believe it to be true and make it happen.

The mind is everything. What you think you become. -Budda

There is more and more research popping up every day that shows a focus on the connection of the gut and the brain. There is a reason people use the phrase 'I have a gut feeling about something' it is literally true. That is where the gut nickname 'second brain' comes from. It can significantly affect your mood and mental state. Studies have revealed that 70% of the neurons outside the brain and spinal cord are located in the gut. The connection between those neurons and the central nervous system is known as the gut-brain axis, or gut-brain connection. This is a two-way communication channel that transmits information from the brain directly to the intestines and vice versa.

Having a healthy gut should be more to you than a lack of heartburn or bloating. The gut health knowledge will become central to your entire health and connected to everything that happens in your body. Therefore when chronic health problems arise you will know to start by fixing the health of the gut first.

There is a connection between gut health and mental health, and what we do know is that drugs, particularly antibiotics, are often destroying the good gut flora and causing dysbiosis, or imbalance in the gut microbiome. Antibiotics save countless lives, but studies show that at least 30% of antibiotics prescribed today are unnecessary. Doing this can disturb the gut flora and lead to antibiotic resistance.

With all the variety of things that can wreak havoc on our gut health some people may feel hopeless and resolve to the false belief that they will always have health issues. They may think that it seems impossible to heal the gut and restore their bodies to optimal health. The body does not heal overnight, but with patience and proper changes, including exercise, diet, and supplementation (including probiotics, prebiotics, and enzymes) it is entirely possible to restore the body to a much healthier you. You can restore the full health of your gastrointestinal system, which can have a major impact, for the positive, on your entire body. Your mood, memory, immune system, everything from the top of your head to the bottoms of your feet will start having the right kind of bacteria that tells your brain that it is okay to feel good again.

People who lack Gut-Brain education can suffer for years looking for answers, Kristin shares how she struggled with pain and discomfort only to be told it was 'normal' after a traumatic event.

My entire life I suffered from migraines, severe cramping, and heavy bleeding during my periods. I also had several ovarian cysts. I just dealt with it because I figured that was how my body just was.

Two days into the new year of 2014 we were on vacation in Arizona visiting some of my husband's family. Like anyone at that time of year, we were excited for what the New Year would bring. We had found out a few weeks earlier that we were expecting our second child. The due date was Labor Day, of all days.

I woke up that New Year's morning with some bleeding and a sinking feeling that something was not right. The bleeding was not really that bad and I did not have any cramping. So, we went about the day hoping everything would be OK.

About 5:00 that night I was holding my daughter and opening the fridge to get her some milk. A pain hit and I quickly handed my daughter to my husband and hurried to the room where we were staying. I did not make it to the bed, however.

After collapsing on the floor the rest of the night was a haze of pain. My husband and his brothers got me to the

Emergency Room and after an ultrasound the doctor told us that I had a tubal pregnancy that ruptured.

They needed to do surgery to remove the damaged tube, repair the internal bleeding, and take the baby. I was devastated. Not only was I losing my baby but, I wondered if I would ever be able to get pregnant again.

When I woke up they told me I had lost so much blood I was borderline for needing a transfusion. After the miscarriage everything got worse, including having constant dizziness, fatigue, and constipation.

Six months later I was still suffering. I told my doctor that I did not feel right. I was told that, due to my traumatic miscarriage, it would take twelve to eighteen months to recover.

We got pregnant again and so the way I felt was chalked-up to the pregnancy. I was so dizzy all the time I could not take care of my other child.

After the baby was born, he would wake up in the night and I would Ping-Pong down the hall and sit on the floor with him to nurse because I was too dizzy and scared that I would hurt him if I tried to carry him anywhere. There were days when the headaches were so severe I could only make it from my bed to the couch.

A year after my little boy was born I still felt like crap. That summer we were on a trip to St. George with my husband's brother and some of his friends. I was sitting pool-side with my brother-in-law's friend, while everyone else went to Zion's National Park to hike the Subway trail. I could not go because of my health issues and she was benched due to a thyroid surgery just a week before the trip.

We were getting to know each other while watching the kids swim in the pool. We were exchanging health issue stories when she told me about some gut health supplements she had just started taking and how they had helped her more *than anything else ever had. Honestly, I did not think too much of it because I had tried supplements before and nothing had helped.*

So, I politely listened with a smile and a nod. A week after we got back from the trip she called me up and invited me to come and learn more about the gut health products she had been taking.

She offered to pick me up and buy me dinner. I figured I would go because hey, it was a night out and a free meal. After hearing her friend explain more about the supplements they were using I thought, 'I have nothing to lose... At least in a couple months when they do not work, just like everything else has not worked, I can at least get my money back.'

Two days into taking the supplements the dizziness was lessening. After week one, no more headaches and no more dizziness. I had not pooped so much in my entire life! After not being able to poop for a year and a half, it was awesome! I had more energy and I did not even want to drink soda or eat candy.

Month three and four, I realized my periods were somewhat on a schedule. After losing a fallopian tube my periods had been anywhere from thirty-two to forty-eight days apart with heavy bleeding and cramping like I had never had before. Here I was having much less bleeding, hardly any cramps, and NO migraines. Not even a headache.

Month six, I was down twenty pounds and feeling great! We found out we were expecting a baby again and I was excited to see what differences my gut health supplements would make with a pregnancy. I had been fairly sick with my daughter and with my son I was sick until at least twenty-five weeks along.

This time I was barely sick and it only lasted about ten weeks. My gums had bled the whole time I was previously pregnant and this time, not at all. I was still tired but, not that bad. My first period after having the baby was not nearly as bad as my first one after the other pregnancies and I did not lose my hair by the handfuls this time around.

I am two and a half years into taking my gut health supplements and I still see how much it is helping to heal my body! There have been a few times when I get out of the habit of taking my daily regiment and I notice a difference for sure. My husband has started taking my supplements and is seeing differences with his health as well. Our kids take amazing kids gut health chewable vitamins and our seven-year-old daughter is on the gut health supplements to help her with some gut issues that she has suffered with.

I am SO blessed and forever thankful that my friend was courageous enough to share her story with me and invite me to learn more about gut health. The changes it has made for my family have really changed everything for us. I can actually spin circles in the backyard with my kids! I can take care of my family! I can take charge of my health and my life.

These supplements have not been a cure-all. I still have off days and sometimes I am 'Zombie Mommy' with occasional sick kids, but every day since starting the gut health supplements is far more better than any day before I took them.

How It All Connects

Digestion, mood, health, and even the way people think are being linked to the Gut-Brain connection. Let's dive in a little more to see how it all connects together.

The Enteric Nervous System (ENS) is about 100 million or so nerve cells that oversee the function of the gastrointestinal tracts. The main role of the ENS is to control digestion. In controlling the digestion it communicates back and forth with the brain as to the overall health of the body's gut which in turn relates directly to its immune system.

The connection between gut health and mental health has been known for some time. Individuals who suffer from gut issues like Celiac disease, Irritable Bowel Syndrome (IBS) or leaky gut are far more likely to also suffer from autoimmune disease and mental health issues, including depression and anxiety. Symptoms related to poor gut health can be as obvious as abdominal pain, bloating, reflux, and flatulence, or less obvious symptoms like headaches, fatigue, joint pain, and a weakened immune system.

When the gut becomes irritated or inflamed, which usually happens when the body is trying to digest foods that are overly processed or they have sensitivity to, the ENS signals the body's Central Nervous System (CNS). When this happens the body triggers the mood changes. With mood changes the digestive function may also affect certain cognitive functions, like memory, sometimes known as brain fog, or thinking skills.

On a positive side, gut health can also impact mental health and mood in a beneficial way. The type of food you eat can have a huge positive effect on the functions of the brain. When the gut is healthy, the brain is happy. Certain bacteria found in the gut can work to help heal and protect the brain in the long term.

Most Americans do have an unhappy brain and an unhealthy gut, due to the processed, sugary and fatty foods that the average American diet is filled with. With this diet the gut becomes damaged over time and less functional. Diets that are filled with simple carbohydrates are severely damaging to the brain. These diets allow the bad bacteria in the gut to grow exponentially. This type of gut-damaging diet has been linked to mental health issues ranging from headaches and ADHD to depression and dementia.

Right now you are thinking of someone you know that fits right into this mold of poor food choices and how it is resulting in their current health situation.

It is not their fault (well it kind of is from a lack of education) but really, there are no lessons in gut health to educate people on the damage they are doing with their poor food choices. In school the basic food pyramid is taught along with a lesson on calories in and calories out. Maybe even a little education on exercise, but gut health is not a top choice in education or even a choice at all.

Most people do not stop to take a look at the 'real damage' that has been done until a health concern or disease pops up and they are forced to make a change. Usually a doctor tells them they have a disease or blood work comes back abnormal or high. Then they stop and think about their health and wonder how it all went downhill. They probably think the diagnosis is just bad luck and not that it is actually a result of choices made in their own life style.

While searching for solutions to her health issues Natalie, a registered nurse from Arizona, learned about the Gut-Brain connection. She realized the 3 key elements to healing the body were improving gut health, decreasing inflammation in the body and balancing her blood sugar.

I was tired, not the tired that a nap can fix or a good night's sleep can cure. More like exhausted emotionally, physically, and spiritually to the extreme. I thought it was 'normal' and par for the course since I had been diagnosed with hypothyroidism and Hashimoto's thyroid disease. Anything that required moving was difficult.

There were times where I would lay on the couch for hours because even the thought of getting up was too much. There was a time that I did not want to do activities with my family or go on vacations with my family because I knew I could not be 'all in' because I would be exhausted.

Along with this fatigue came the guilt of feeling lazy, having too much to do, and not having the energy to do it. I felt like a horrible mom and wife.

I had gone to see doctors, many doctors, received good care and a prescription to help! I did my research, I am a nurse, I should have all the answers right?? Things I tried worked for a short time and then went back to 'my' normal.

In addition to the fatigue my list of other issues was extensive: weight gain, GI symptoms, bloating, constipation, pain, frequent migraines, brain fog, balance issues, dizziness, lack of focus and motivation, and all of them were getting worse.

Emotionally I was having new anxiety symptoms that started while my husband was serving in Afghanistan and did not stop after he came home. This was coupled with bouts of depression. I hated how I felt! Every day I would think to myself, this cannot be normal, there has to be a better way. I wanted to be better, healthy, happy, for my 3 girls, for my husband, for me! I wanted my life back.

Being a Registered Nurse for 18 years at that point I started to do some more research. I focused more in finding solutions vs finding things to treat my symptoms. I also started praying. Pretty good combination huh!? One night when my sister-in-law was visiting she told me she had a friend who is a nurse and she wanted us to check out these supplements for the gut.

My first thought was, 'I have tried so many things, no way.' But when she started saying things like 'improved gut health, better sleep, MORE energy and reducing systemic inflammation,' my curiosity was peaked. Then I thought, what the heck, what have I got to lose?? I will give it a shot. So I did! I jumped in, with both feet and I am so SO grateful I did!!

Fast forward two and a half years, and that long list of issues I was having are all GONE! I finally feel like myself again. Do I still have some bad days, sure… thank you autoimmune disease!!! BUT, even my bad days now pale in comparison to my best days before!

Secret 6

What the Heck is Leaky Gut

What the heck is leaky gut, and how do you know if you have it?

In an ever increasing world of natural health you have probably heard the term leaky gut, but you may not know what it really is. Depending on who you ask you may get a different answer every time.

'Leaky gut syndrome is something of a medical mystery. From an MD's standpoint, it's a very gray area' said Rudolph Bedford, MD, a gastroenterologist at Providence Saint John's Health Center in Santa Monica, California.

I love what Christy shares about healing her leaky gut and not stressing over the holidays. When she first started working on healing her body, her level of Candida was one of the worst cases that her functional medicine doctor had ever seen.

When our gut bacteria is out of balance, we feel like crap: Tired, sluggish, sadness, anxiousness, blah-ness, excess, stubborn weight, belly fat, headaches, foggy brain, sugar cravings, sleep problems, soreness, stiff joints, ongoing infections of all kinds, poor immune health, tiredness, skin issues, and ON and ON.

{fun fact: Google 'Candida yeast overgrowth' and ANY symptom, there is a connection}

I found some great natural gut health products that are a simple, easy, and effective way to address the bad bacteria overgrowth in your gut, and repopulate your gut with beneficial bacteria. It is sustainable, and long-term. {Praise the heavens above!}

In the last 2+ years I have lost a whole lot of things, since starting to give my body what it needs to be balanced, and heal itself.

Some of the things I have lost:

Afternoon slumps/naps, sugar cravings, achy body, racing heart, drawn-out sad feelings, belly fat, always being sick, fear of my future health, brain fog, headaches, stomach discomfort, weekly trips to see my Pediatrician with sick babies, sleep issues, breathing struggles, to name a few....

OH! and FIFTY POUNDS.

Not because I take a magic formula that makes my body lose weight, but because I am working with my body to balance it at the root, and keep it balanced. And one of those side-effects is releasing excess weight.

I get it. I used to not really understand. I judged, rolled my eyes, the whole snotty, skeptical girl bit. But DANG am I glad I humbled myself and STUCK with this! It just keeps getting better and better.

I feel freaking fantastic! I want to share a 'celebration' with my friends...Today, it is official. I have lost fat, and several pounds over the holidays!

WHAAA?!?!

This has never happened to me! I have officially reached my lowest weight since having my son almost 2 years ago. And how in the world is it possible to drop weight over the holidays?

UMMM???

It is helpful when you are craving things like brussel sprouts and carrots.

TROOF...I do not really care about that number on the scale. That is not really a thing to me.

What I AM excited about is the indicator it is to me. It tells me my body is healthy and whole. It tells me that it is not about black and white thinking, all or nothing. It is the magic of the gray area. It tells me that listening to my body's cues, and following them works. It tells me that by working with my body to heal the roots of my health, those branches are thriving too. I am reaching my weight management goals as a side benefit - yasssss.

You see, I am not on a mission to lose weight (of course I love the idea of trimming up!) I AM on a mission to be as healthy and thriving from the inside out as I can be. To take the very best care of my body that I can. For my sake, my family's sake and so I can show up in my life the way I was designed to. To also be balanced, and not obsess about extremes in the process. You better believe I had some yummy morsels over the holidays! I also enjoyed some spinach artichoke dip and pecan pie...MM HMM.

I literally do not crave sugar anymore so, if I want a treat, I can have a bite or two and then I feel done. I stop. And this is magic. It is that magical, UN-perfectionist gray area. It is balance. And to know that I can live this way and maintain this life style is sooo exciting to me!- It is empowering!

Causes of Leaky Gut

Leaky gut, or leaky gut syndrome, sometimes called intestinal permeability, occurs when the intestinal wall becomes irritated and stops working the way it should.

Think of the intestinal wall like a piece of tightly woven material. Normally this wall is so tightly woven it provides a protective barrier that absorbs particles from toxins, foods, and microorganisms. When leaky gut occurs this mesh becomes looser and not so tight. The holes in the mesh become bigger which allows the particles to 'leak' through instead of being absorbed. When these particles leak through they can make their way into the bloodstream. It is a mysterious condition in a sense that it can cause mysterious health issues.

There is no official test to diagnose leaky gut and no way of telling if health issues are caused by leaky gut alone.

If you have leaky gut you probably also have many other health issues as well.

So how does the tightly woven mesh of the gut become weak? The exact cause is not known but has been linked to inflammation in the gut.

Leaky gut has been linked to inflammation conditions such as Celiac disease, Crohn's disease, and inflammatory bowel disease. Leaky gut has also been linked to irritants in the stomach from NSAID pain relievers, alcohol, and antibiotics. Inflammatory foods like gluten, sugar, dairy, or other foods that are hard to digest may also irritate the stomach and lead to inflammation in the gut.

When particles get leaked into the blood stream the body will see them as a foreign object or invaders in the body. The body will trigger the immune system to attack them. When the body attacks these particles it creates more inflammation. A vicious cycle of problems related to leaky gut and inflammation continues on and on and never clears up.

Dr. Taz Bhatia, integrative health expert and author of the *21 Day Belly Fix* explains how over time inflammation caused by leaky gut syndrome can trigger problems. Problems like bloating, gas, cramps, psoriasis, eczema, and allergies. He says. 'It could also lead to fatigue, unexplained pains, or even depression. When food particles make their way into the blood stream instead of getting properly digested, the body is less able to absorb nutrients- including vitamins B and D, magnesium, and certain amino acids that can impact mood and energy levels.'

If you experience conditions that relate to leaky gut syndrome it may be time to talk to your doctor about it. Testing for Celiac disease, Crohn's disease, or irritable bowel syndrome may be an option to look at.

Marjorie, from Hawaii, shares about how it is never too late in life to start working on healing your gut.

I am currently seventy and retired in October 2015. I had a demanding job managing staff in a Medical Management Department. On top of that, I had to commute daily and my job was sedentary with lots of meetings and projects.

I neglected my health for quite some time and had some health issues that I did not pay attention to. It was not anything that I would go to the doctor for. I am not one to go to the doctor very often. Besides, the usual MD solution is to write a prescription and come back in two weeks.

I also had intestinal issues. . . lots of bloating and diarrhea after eating a meal. Sometimes I would eat and twenty to thirty minutes later I would need to go to the nearest bathroom. I ignored this too, even though it was embarrassing and I knew it was not normal.

In December 2015, I went to Kauai to watch my daughter's children for a week. That was really hard. My body ached all over and my joints hurt. I was overweight and had little energy. Sometimes at night I could not sleep just because my body ached.

I usually had daily headaches and took pain relievers almost daily to manage the headaches. I was a grazer also. . . would piece all day. . . especially on sweet things. My daughter had told me about some natural gut health supplements and had me try them, but I was not really into it! I was trying to be nice to her because she believed in it so much.

At Christmas, I was going to Kauai again but did not feel well enough to go early so I flew over on Christmas Day, somewhat recovered from nagging back pain which I thought was a spasm (turned out to be facet joint problem). During the time I was there, I felt really terrible.

My daughter sat me down and said, 'Mom, you are unhealthy! You have got to get serious about this!' I told her I was not unhealthy. . . I did not have any diagnosed, chronic conditions. Yes, I was overweight but healthy eating and moderate exercise should take care of that. . . if I had the energy to do it!

So I decided to really take my supplements the way I should have and do moderate exercise and commit to better health from the inside out. I made sure I drank my water daily. . .I used to hate water. . .it always needed to be sweetened.

I had never really taken supplements seriously before because I never felt any different. About two to three months into my routine I added omegas.

So what are my results. . .

•I have lost forty pounds and gone from a size fourteen to a size eight. I never kept track of the inches and I am not usually one that weighs much.

•I lost all craving for sugar which was one of the first things I noticed. I listen to my body and eat when I am hungry but I honestly crave carrots, hummus, boiled eggs, and salads. . . good stuff. That does not mean I do not eat a cookie or have a piece of pie when I want. It just means I do not really care if I have any.

•I sleep a much deeper sleep than I ever did before. I actually sleep.

•My bloating and diarrhea have resolved. I do not have to worry if I go out for lunch that I will need to be close to a bathroom in 20-30 minutes. That is freedom!

•*I rarely have a headache anymore and that is miraculous.*

•*My all over body aches and joint pain has lessened so much that it does not keep me awake and it keeps improving. It does not hold me back from doing anything I want to do.*

•*I do a brisk one hour walk daily and feel so much more internal stamina. That is the only way I can explain it. I have energy to do everything I want to do.*

•*I do not crave any kind of daytime naps. Even if I wanted to take a nap I cannot.*

•*When I had a recent physical exam, my HDL was 85 and my triglycerides were 67. Awesome numbers for an old lady.*

In short, I feel healthier and stronger than I have in many years. I have been taking my gut health supplements for thirty months now and plan to continue the rest of my life.

I have loved how this is not a diet or anything complicated. It is just giving my body the nutrients it needs that it was not getting before, and then listening to my body give me the cues I need to eat appropriately and exercise. I truly feel that I can enjoy the rest of my life and age the way God intended.

I am not headed for a life full of prescriptions and doctor visits and all the stuff usually associated with growing older. I am grateful my daughter stuck with me for so long and got me on the right path.

I had just accepted that I was getting older and was going to feel the way I felt. I was wrong. We don't have to accept the status quo or just get another prescription!

Secret 7

How To Stop the Leak in Your Gut

Things you can do to help leaky gut symptoms naturally is cleaning up your diet. For some people gluten, processed sugar, and dairy are tougher to digest and can trigger inflammation. If you cut out these foods (even temporarily as your body heals) it helps reduce inflammation. If you cut out these foods for at least six to twelve weeks you give your body and gut a little time to heal and stop new inflammation from developing.

Once the gut starts to heal you may be able to introduce some of the foods back into your diet, in small quantities. You may start to feel so good without them that you may want to leave the foods out of your diet all together. You may decide the sluggish feelings are not worth it and never add those foods back.

Husbands can really tell a difference in their wives when they feel better and have more energy. Shaun shares his experience with his wife in regard to how he feels now that she has been healing her leaky gut.

First, my wife has always been all about healthy remedies, healthy eating and living right. She has always battled with weight issues. I thought some of that was genetics for her. I also thought a lot of her troubles came from having kids.

She has always been able to run long distances without stopping. She could go out and run for hours. Even when she was running every day, she struggled with weight and gut issues.

She has had allergies since she was a kid. She has a long list of issues she has dealt with (sometimes the symptom list did not seem real). What I did not know was that she has battled depression for years. She hid it well – even from me. Two years ago, before she discovered some natural gut health supplements, she was having more emotional problems that I did not expect or know how to handle.

She found these gut health supplements through some friends and from her research she knew a lot of the ingredients and products were really good. She actually decided to order the products without telling me. She told me about them after she had been taking them a while because she was feeling better. I took her word for it, but the first couple things I personally noticed was that her mood improved greatly and she had more energy.

She has always been a night owl and hated the mornings. I noticed one morning that she got up before my alarm clock went off (never happened before). She got up and started doing laundry. I thought maybe I had made her mad or something. The truth was she was rested and ready to take on the day – so she just woke up! She did not need to take a nap after those long runs any more. This is a regular occurrence now – almost two years later.

My wife is optimistic about life again. She has dropped dress sizes and a few pounds. She has lost more inches than pounds. She does not lose her hair like she used to. She has more energy at home and when working out. I cannot imagine her without these products. It has made such a difference for us as a couple as well as for her physically and emotionally.

She has also had a great experience building her health business. She is becoming a better leader every day. She has been super supportive of me and my business. We help each other now. I lost my job last year and we have been through some crazy financial trials this last year. I KNOW that my old wife could not have made it through this last year of stress without her gut being healthy. She has been so optimistic and supportive. It has been great working with her on her business and mine.

My wife started the kids on the gut health products after she took them a while. I was the last in our house to start taking them. I always thought I was pretty healthy. Since taking certain products myself, I am down about fifteen pounds. I have been able to handle stress better. I sleep better and feel better. These products have been a blessing in our lives.

I can tell you that people have different experiences using gut health supplements. Some because they do not take them regularly. Some because they have different problems than you and I might have. Some because they do not stick with it long enough. But I can tell you that they help. For most people, it takes a while for their bodies to correct. But for those who stick with it – it is worth it. These are not cure-all drugs. It is just a tool to help your body work the way it should.

Getting proper supplements in your body can also help heal the gut. Moderate exercise and hydrating the body with the proper amount of water will also help the body to achieve better health. Milk, soda, sport drinks, and juices do not count as water for the body. The body needs good old clean and pure water to stay hydrated. 1-2 glasses of water are not enough to stay hydrated.

There are many apps and calculators to figure out what your body needs. A good rule of thumb is to take your body weight and divide it in half. Take that number and that is how many ounces you should drink. So if you weight 100lbs then 50oz of water is a good amount to drink. There are some people who have health issues that may not be able to drink that much and there may be other reasons, like exercise where you may need to add in more. Talking to your doctor to find the right amount of water for you is ideal.

Increasing fiber intake with gut supporting fiber and cutting out processed and refined foods will help the gut heal. Eating whole foods is best. If it has a label on it, avoid it.

If 75% of your plate is vegetables and plant-based foods you are probably getting high fiber foods and your gut will thank you.

Eat good fats like omega's and monounsaturated fats like extra-virgin olive oil. These good fats will help decrease inflammation and give good bacteria a chance to flourish. If you are not a fan of fishy omega's you can get a plant-based omega that is vegetarian. You will also want to supplement with a good probiotic or several good probiotic strains. A good probiotic will help reduce inflammation and increase the growth of good bacteria.

Coconut oil is anti-inflammatory with great benefits. Coconut oil and coconut butter contain fabulous fat-burning MCT's (Medium chain triglyceride). MCT oils may be linked to weight loss benefits as well. Cut out the inflammatory fats like vegetable oil. Nuts and seeds provide your gut with prebiotics and feed your healthy bacteria. Also adding in fermented foods such as sauerkraut, kimchi, tempeh, and miso help your good bacteria multiply because of the amount of good probiotics in them.

Hannah, 23 from Utah, talks about how she developed an eating disorder from issues relating to her poor gut health.

Seven years after recovering from the restrictive eating disorder that stemmed from my horrible tummy issues, my mind was healed. My body, however, was not.

As a freshman in high school, I found myself struggling with horrible stomach pains and completely miserable. It led me to restricting my intake from 500 calories a day, to nothing at all to escape the pain. I lost 25% of my body weight, was hospitalized, and started the journey of healing.

I went to countless therapy and pediatric appointments. I gained the weight back and I learned the tools I needed to cope with these restrictive thoughts. My body reacted the same way to food though, and because of my unhealthy restrictive tendencies, I was not allowed to restrict anything (per my doctor) to find the source.

Fast forward to April 2017! I had woken up late for work, in horrible tummy pain, and had anxious feelings. 'Something needs to change.' I thought to myself. SOMETHING!

A few days later I saw my friend posting on social media about some natural gut health supplements. I had never heard of gut health before. I reached out, ordered the products, and started on it religiously.

I was lucky, and saw results within two weeks when I realized I had not taken my stomach medicine since I started. And then I started waking up before my alarm. And then I fell asleep quickly at night.

My tummy was not hurting me anymore!! I could drink milkshakes and eat cereal and eat red meat without the consequences. And I have not swallowed one of those little green tummy pills since. My husband Sam has also lost 30 lbs. on the natural gut health products and sustained it. So amazing.

I am so so thankful.

Secret 8

How You Are Murdering Your Good Bacteria;

Stop Killing Yourself

We have talked a little bit about how the food you eat can cause havoc on the gut microbiome. These food choices are killing good bacteria and usually make you feel guilty and dampen your mood. You may feel the effects immediately or over time. We have all heard the term 'hangry' well it has everything to do with the gut. It is when you are hungry and angry at the same time.

Some foods might not be the smartest choice to eat. Refined carbohydrates in recent years have been the front of foods to avoid. These carbohydrates have a reputation of being fat-promoting, nutrient-lacking and it is true.

Using data from the Woman's Health Initiative, which is tracking more than 70,000 woman, the researchers 'found that the higher a woman's blood sugar rose after eating sugar and refined grains, the higher her risk of depression.' In this study published in the *American Journal of Clinical Nutrition*, the researchers also found the reverse to be true 'A diet in whole grains and produce actually lowers a woman's risk of depression.'

James Wythe, from Poole, England, a fully qualified Health Coach and Food Blogger shares his story of how he used nutrition to heal his body.

I want to give you an insight into the main reasons why I decided to change my lifestyle and what motivated me to share this with more people.

It all started when I fell ill in December 2010 just after completing my sports science BS (bachelor of science) Degree at Bournemouth University (where I was playing golf for the University and also the Dorset County 1st Team).

I thought my illness was just a touch of food poisoning but for some reason I did not recover and the symptoms just seemed to get worse and worse. I tried to push through this but reached a point where I had to be rushed into the hospital for a suspected brain tumor. I had several brain scans but I was so weak at that point having lost nearly three stone (42 pounds) in weight that I could not eat, drink or even stand up!

On my third trip to the hospital I was kept in for eleven days. I was tested for everything they could think of, however all the tests came back 'normal.' At that point I had also become hypersensitive to more and more of the medication they were giving me. I also had a severe allergic reaction and developed sensitivity to light, smells and certain foods. The doctors were unable to give any diagnosis apart from saying that I had some kind of viral infection, so they just sent me home and told me to rest and take it easy for a while.

I did go home and rest, unfortunately I did not recover or feel any better; in fact I just got worse. I was bed bound, unable to stand up or walk by myself. I could not watch TV or look at my phone as I was extremely sensitive to the light which would give me awful headaches but to make matters worse, I suffered with severe insomnia often going days without any sleep at all. This made it impossible to see my friends and made me feel really isolated.

After multiple attempts to get help from the doctors they finally, after nearly six months, diagnosed me with M.E. (Myalgic Encephalomyelitis) also known as CFS (Chronic

Fatigue Syndrome). I was told there was no 'cure' and all I could do was rest and wait.

I started to follow some social media pages about M.E to gain more knowledge and came across a page called Let's Do It For M.E (LDIFME) who were raising money for UK charity Invest in ME to do extensive research into the illness particularly into the gut.

Over the next few months I contacted all friends and family members and managed to raise £3000 (The charity raised funds to match the donation making a total of £6000) towards the research which really helped them hit the £100,000 goal they had set. If you wish to donate to this charity or find out more about M.E then go to http://ldifme.org/foundation-research-project/.

My parents, especially my mum, were amazing throughout this time not leaving a leaf unturned in order to find out how they could help me recover. I needed full time care and my mum had to stay with me twenty four hours a day for several months.

We also got in touch with the M.E. clinic in Wareham to visit and to try to help me cope with my illness. During that horrible time my mum started reading everything she could in order to find alternative ways to make me feel better.

She booked a nutritionist and also arranged for a Bowen specialist (Bowen is a holistic remedial body technique that works on the soft connective tissue of the body) to see me at my house and try to improve my situation. It was interesting as the nutritionist I was seeing at that time had also suffered from M.E. many years earlier and therefore could relate to my story, she told me to immediately cut gluten and dairy from my diet which my mum and I had already talked about prior to that.

I had always had a pretty balanced diet and never feasted on typical takeaway food but we had not considered looking more carefully at what I was really eating. That was the first step into changing my diet and nutrition along with taking supplements, some of which came from America specifically designed for M.E. sufferers.

At first this was a major change from eating a normal balanced diet to really having to think about exactly what to eat and what that food actually contained. My mum also had to change the way she prepared food but after just a short while this became less of a challenge and actually became the norm.

I was also very lucky to get closer to a girl called Luise, she had heard through mutual friends about what I was going through and started coming to visit me. It was very hard for me and Luise as I was not able to even talk on some days let alone sit up or be a nice host, however she never failed to come and see me and that is when our relationship developed into something more serious.

Luise also really helped my parents in sharing the hard work and in particular has supported my mum during the long journey towards my continued recovery.

Around six months after taking special supplements, sticking rigidly to a new nutritional plan and having Bowen treatment, I slowly started to gain a little energy. I managed to walk outside of my bedroom along the landing by myself which sounds like a small thing but for me at the time was a huge achievement.

Over the next few months I was able to walk downstairs, but the effort would really tire me out and I was not able to attempt this again for a few days or even up to a week.

Over the next few months I set myself challenges and pushed myself a little bit harder, so I would try and walk to the gate at the end of the drive just twenty yards each way which seemed like a marathon to me. The first time I stepped outside it felt extremely odd to me as I had been confined to the four walls in my bedroom for over 6 months, everything felt so unexplainably large and I found it overwhelming.

A year later I was still very much bed bound but occasionally I could be driven to a local shop and to walk around for a few minutes before going home and retiring back to bed. A few months later I also managed to finally take Luise on our first official date (well actually Luise took me out) which felt like a real milestone for us both!

After two years of being confined to my bed for the majority of the time and recovering at a very slow pace, and after long discussions with my parents, Luise and I managed to move into a flat together in Bournemouth. Luise was still at Bournemouth University and also working part time so I was home alone more often than not and had to again push myself in order to feed and care for myself.

During that time I really discovered that I liked researching and preparing healthy and fresh food as well as looking into easy and quick gluten and dairy free dishes as I did not have the energy to cook for hours.

Another year had passed and I started seeing a local nutritionist who really helped me to clean up my diet and to cut out processed sugars as much as possible. I started reading many alternative cook books which inspired me a lot and helped build my passion to cook and eat and live as healthily as possible.

Now, I am at a stage where I can look back and see what a huge impact food has had in my recovery, the more I clean up my diet the better my energy levels become. I keep discovering more and more ways to eat healthily but without making it super complicated. Luise still supports me with this all the time even though I leave the kitchen in a complete mess nearly every day.

I am not unique and there are many people that have suffered or are suffering from similar health problems. Those people, along with their friends and loved ones find it really frustrating and painful to try and find help and support.

Healthy living is one of the ways I have found that works and I hope that sharing my experiences may offer a way forward.

This is just a small look into my illness and the way that I have adapted, learned and moved forward towards a healthy lifestyle and I am happy to provide more information if anyone has any questions or wants to talk more about M.E.

You can follow Healthy James at healthylivingjames. co.uk or grab his free ebook at healthylivingjames.co.uk/free-ebook

Foods to Avoid

Processed sugar is another food to stay as far away from as you can. Processed sugar contributes to a higher risk of depression. A diet high in processed sugar will increase levels of inflammation in the body and the brain. Sugar is the root of chronic inflammation. If you want to lower levels of chronic inflammation; eliminate sugar from your diet. This in turn will also help your mood.

When people want to stay away from sugar they usually turn to artificial sweeteners. This is even worse than processed sugar. Can I repeat that? Artificial sweeteners are worse than sugar!!! Especially if you have depression, please stay away.

Artificial sweeteners are a synthetic foreign substance and the body does not know what to do with it. These foreign substances can have a big impact on your serotonin levels and reduce that happy hormone in the brain.

Stay away from Trans fats. These are not the good fats. These are the fats that are artery-clogging and can increase your risk of depression by as much as 48% according to a study published in *PLOS ONE*. The good fats like olive oil can actually lower the risk of a number of health conditions, so if you are going to consume oil, consume the better choice.

Processed foods are another big NO, NO. These are creeping into our diets more and more. With food 'ready to eat' and 'simple to make' it is no surprise that this category can have all the other bad choices inside it. Our body needs digestive enzymes to break down food. When you eat whole foods, like fresh fruits and veggies, they have natural digestive enzymes in them. When you eat processed foods your body has to pull enzymes from somewhere else, usually leaving an enzyme deficiency somewhere else in the body. These foods can lead to an increase in the risk of depression. If it has a label, it is likely processed, so choose to eat foods that have not been altered or created by man.

Secret 9

How Your Lifestyle Impacts Your Health

Throughout the year's term like 'Chi, qi, life force, and soul' were names given to energy to describe the energy or life force in our bodies and the well-being of our bodies.

Civilizations have been healing their bodies naturally with this energy, but somehow over the years we have strayed away from it. More and more people are trying to get back to their roots and heal their bodies in a natural way.

Part of this disconnect over the years has come from our lifestyle changes and modern technology.

We live in a society that discourages 'potty talk' and thinks it is not socially acceptable to talk about what comes out of our bodies.

'What happens in the bathroom should stay in the bathroom' is a common thing taught to kids when they are young. Through the years as people have learned to not talk about their waste, they do not even know what is 'normal' anymore. Someone who poops once a day may think they are constipated because they are not pooping after every meal and someone who poops once a week may think they are 'just fine or regular' since that is what they have always done.

When you ask kids about how often they poop or what it looks like they get embarrassed and do not want to talk about it. If a child talks about poop it usually is in jokes or in the content of 'being naughty.'

The media tells us that if we have bathroom issues it is embarrassing and we need to get rid of the issues immediately.

Go see a doctor or take a pill and 'fix it' as soon as possible. The waste our body produces is sending us messages and by shutting down those messages we are only making the issues worse. The media wants us to think we should shut it down, turn it off, cover it up, and move on. We should not have to be inconvenienced with these issues any longer.

Our poop can actually communicate a lot about our health. We need to learn to be more open about it. We should be making it more a part of our daily communication. Our children should be able to talk openly about it. That way they learn it is part of health education and part of their well-being.

If your body is not disposing of waste properly, if your poop is too loose, too hard, you have cramps, bloating, gas, or you are uncomfortable, your body is trying to tell you something and you should listen to it right away.

There are many environmental things or outside forces that make us feel violated that can also affect our gut health. Many of these things are never discussed. Physical violence, sexual abuse, verbal and emotional abuse can all shut down a person's ability to listen to their body, see signs, or receive messages from the gut. In most cases people just shut down, ignore messages and close them in to forget what they have gone through.

There are also traumas to the body that can affect gut health. Traumas such as surgery, pregnancy, abortion, painful menstrual cramps can all affect your gut health and cause you to ignore the messages coming from your gut.

Society also tells you that if you are an intelligent person you can explain away the issues and not listen to your 'gut feelings.'

Your lifestyles which include what you eat, how much you eat, how much you exercise, if you sit at a desk all day, or if you are stressed to the max with life and problems, all affect the health of your gut.

Do you ignore these messages and just think of the issues as an 'inconvenience' that you need a doctor to take away? Are you really listening and realizing that what you do and your daily actions are affecting your gut health? Do you need to stop and listen?

People do not take notice of their gut until the issues become worse and start to affect their health. Once their health is affected, they still want a doctor to give them a pill instead of taking a closer look at their own lives and how they have been treating their body for years.

I have seen people go in for surgeries and have organs removed instead of listening to the messages and trying to find the root cause of the issue. If it bothers them they would rather just 'take it out' than worry about making a lifestyle change or correcting choices they have made.

Utah Pediatrician Jessika W. shares how gut health supplements have helped her improve her energy, deal with constipation, and lose unwanted weight.

I am a wife, a mom of four kids under the age of nine, a full time pediatrician, and gut health supplement lifer!

I have been using a great line of natural gut health supplements since July 2016. I started using them when I decided to participate in a seven day trial of one product.

For a few years, but intensely a few months before that, I had been researching gut health and magnesium supplementation after some continuing medical education lectures that I attended about gut health, and the impact our gut microbiome has on our weight and overall health.

My husband's cousin had been sharing information about some great supplements she had been using that focused on gut health, regulating blood sugar, and decreased inflammation in her body, so after looking into it, I quickly realized the supplements were exactly what I was looking for. I knew I needed to get my gut healthy to fix my issues, and these supplements offered exactly what I wanted!

I started taking these supplements when my fourth baby was about five and a half weeks old. I was sick and tired of feeling sluggish, heavy, grumpy, and hangry all the time. I was constantly looking for my next sugar fix to keep me going. I had very hard stools, even though I was taking daily stool softeners since I was pregnant with my first child. (Six years of daily stool softeners!) I gained ten pounds between each pregnancy, so I was certainly overweight.

I was 'too busy' taking care of everyone else at home and at work, so I did not bother taking care of myself. Pretty much the only thing I was doing right was drinking lots of water! So, I decided to jump in full steam and commit to these new supplements in an effort to take care of myself.

Within a few days I noticed my sugar cravings were nearly gone. I was not feeling hangry all the time. Within a week and a half, I was off my stool softeners and have not taken one since! YEAH! I started to notice I was moving more and playing with my kids instead of just watching them. I just felt better. I felt lighter and happier. I was sleeping better, even with a newborn!

After three months, I knew I wanted to keep taking these products forever. That was the first time I stepped on the scale. I was down twelve pounds. All of my pants were too loose. Really the only thing I had intentionally changed was taking the gut health supplements.

I was naturally eating better because my blood sugar was balanced, and my sugar cravings stopped. I was not carrying around full bowels and excessive Candida like before. I was moving my body more but not intentionally exercising.

Since then, I have begun exercising occasionally, but it is still an area I struggle with. I am working on eating better, but I still have a ways to go. In the first ten months I lost thirty pounds. I have not lost any weight since then, but I have purchased new work clothes twice because I'm still losing inches! I sometimes tell people I would not even care if I had only lost one pound if I still felt as good as I feel! Gut health supplements have changed my life and I will NEVER look back!

I started on a combination of gut health supplements and probiotics, but I have also began Omega supplements, more varieties of probiotics strains, and methylated vitamins. I just weaned my nearly twenty-one-month-old from nursing and felt very comfortable as both a mom and pediatrician taking these products the whole time while nursing.

Sleep

Gut health is linked in the quality and timing of your sleep through your sleep-wake cycles, or your circadian rhythm. When you have higher levels of Candida and other "bad" bacteria it is a direct correlation to sleep problems and fatigue. An unbalanced gut can perpetuate sleep problems.

Your circadian rhythms regulate the gut immune responses so when your circadian rhythms are misaligned it can lead to an unbalanced gut microbiome even more.

This rhythm disruption of the circadian timing of sleep leads to a more broad range of health issues such as obesity, inflammation, metabolic disease, and mood disorders. This is very important to know if you are someone that works on a night shift or other schedules that might effect when the body would normally sleep.

Stress

The health of your gut has a direct relation to how your body handles stress.

Think of stress like a flashlight, when you need it, you can turn it on. When you are finished with that flashlight you can shut it off. If you do not shut the flashlight off then you can burn out the battery. Compare this flashlight to stress, when you have a little stress it can be good for you, but too much and you burn out.

Imagine you are walking down the street and a large dog jumps out from behind a bush. Your stress fight or flight level kicks in to let your body know that you need to do something to get to safety. You can then run, walk, or move out of the way of the dog. Once that situation has returned to normal that stress fight or flight level goes down and you know you are safe.

What happens if you have too much stress in your life and the levels never come down? You can wear out just like the battery. It may even become life threatening to your health to live on such high levels of stress without a down time. As a result you neglect the health of your mind, body, and spirit.

Some stress we have control over and other stress we may not, but we do have control over how we react to stress. You can create a way to handle stress to help your body be healthier. You can start with hope. You can create hope in your life because when you have no hope stress wins. There are always solutions to come up with. If you are unhealthy you can have hope that you can make changes.

You can change your eating habits or add more water to your day. You can start small to improve your exercise, take a walk, that over time turns into a run. Go for a bike ride. Park far away and walk farther or take the stairs wherever you are.

You can also add in supplements. Work with your doctor to make healthy changes in your life. There is always room for improvement and there is always hope. Make a plan and follow through with it.

If you are in an unhealthy situation or environment, make a plan to get help, get out, change a job, or change a relationship. Ask friends and family for help, access community resources for support.

Most people do not realize all the resources that are available within their own community. Do a little research, go to your city office, or ask around. You will find more information and resources than you thought would be available.

There may be circumstances in your life that you have no control over or trials that may just fall upon you. Some people stress over things they have no control over. Let that stress go, do not let it bring you down.

You may not be able to decide what happens to you but you can decide how you will react to how you handle it. Have a positive attitude. Embrace the challenges of life and use whatever resources you have to help you through them.

Open your mind and know the options that are before you. Expect the unexpected. Explore your passion and dreams in life. If there are things bringing you down look and see what can be done to change them.

Make a commitment to yourself that you are important enough to love.

Make a commitment to yourself by making healthy choices because you are worth it. Have hope and stand tall.

You will be surprised that when you are confident in yourself you will be able to handle the stresses that come at you in a much more positive way, and that in turn will keep you healthier.

Courage will now be your best defense against the storm that is at hand- that and such hope as I bring.
-J.R.R. Tolkien, The Return of the King

Tami shares how her poor gut health had impacted her to the point of being in a wheelchair, but with patience and good gut health supplementation she is now walking again.

I would like to share with you why getting my gut healthy has changed my life. In 2008 I was a busy mom to eight children, a foster parent and busy with church responsibilities. I was diagnosed with Multiple Sclerosis (MS). I just felt like I had so much going on I could not possibly live with this debilitating disease. Over the next ten years I battled being in and out of a wheelchair and not able to care for myself let alone my family.

Some of the things that were affected by MS were, eyesight, pain, constipation, headaches, foot drop, loss of balance, fatigue and depression. I gained weight and was in a deep depression. I had read some articles about how getting my gut healthy would help get my body healthy. I was desperate to find something to help me function better. I tried several medications that various doctors had prescribed. I did not find anything that helped me. I had to find something to help me function better. So I quit the medicine I knew was not working for me.

With the things that I had read I knew I had to get my gut healthy. I started by changing the things I was eating, but I struggled to be dedicated to only putting good things in my body. I had heard about some gut health supplements that would help me get my body healthy. I in no way believed that some supplements would help me get healthy. I was wrong. It was much easier to eat good things once I started taking the supplements. I was desperate to feel better. I noticed that several things changed for me. Part of my eyesight returned, I don't need or crave sugar, I quit a three a day soda habit, my hair quit falling out, no more constipation, I gained some strength, I still have some falls but my balance has improved,

I lost some pounds, and I have less fatigue. When it comes to my depression I have had some relief.

Today I have joy in my life. I also have been healthy and strong. I was able to travel to my daughter's house and be there for the delivery of another grandchild. I have also had the opportunity to go stay at my son's house to help take care of my grandkids while my daughter-in-law recovered from a surgery. Even a year ago I would not have been able to do these things. It is all because my gut is healthy and so is the rest of my body.

Secret 10

The Songs Your Organs Are Singing to You

Organs

Every organ in your body has an important role and all affect the health of your gut. Let's go over and explain a few of the organs and how they relate to your overall gut health.

The Mouth: This is where all your food goes in. You take food in and chew to break it down. When you chew you are mixing that food with saliva. The digestive process has already begun as soon as the food enters in the mouth for the first time.

When you chew it is important to chew and chew and chew so that you are breaking food down as much as possible before you swallow it.

Saliva has a job of attacking unwanted viruses, bacteria, and toxins that enter with food into your mouth. There are antibodies in your saliva that attack those toxins and bacteria that have entered without permission. When you chew your food you are also breaking it down for better digestion and absorption. When you break down the food better you have a much greater chance of absorbing the nutrients in that food.

The Stomach: Your stomach is the main organ in your body for digesting and storing your food. When food enters the stomach your brain kicks in and sends digestive enzymes to break it all down. It is important to know that processed foods do not have digestive enzymes and so your body has to pull them from somewhere else to compensate.

There are many things that can slow down the digestive process like depression, sadness, and anger.

Other things like alcohol, stress, and poor food choices can damage the protective lining inside the stomach causing problems such as ulcers (another message from the gut that something is out of balance).

After your stomach has finished the first stage of digestion and after it has also killed off any organisms that may be harmful to the body, it then passes the partially digested food down the small intestine.

When you eat a meal it is best to drink liquids, including water, thirty minutes before or after a meal because the liquids can dilute the digestive enzymes and cause the digestive process to not be as effective as it could be.

The Small Intestine: The small intestine is approximating 25 feet in length (small but not short). The tubing of the small intestine continues the process of separating the nutrients from the food and the toxins. As food passes through the small intestine juices from the pancreas are released to neutralize stomach acids.

This neutralizing process is what protects the lining of the small intestine. Hormones from your blood also trigger the gallbladder to release bile. This bile breaks down fats. This whole process in the small intestine breaks down the food into nutrients that can be absorbed and used by the body.

This absorption is one of the most important steps in the digestive process. The nutrient absorption is vital to the health of the body.

If you are not absorbing nutrients your health will be compromised and you will be at risk for developing health issues.

The usable nutrients are then sent along to the blood stream and down to the liver. Once the liver has received them they are filtered again even more. After filtration the nutrients are released to the body again.

When there is an over use of certain medications, alcohol consumption, poorly digested food, and stress, the lining that is the protective part of the small intestine can be compromised and toxins can leak through into the bloodstream. When this occurs it is known as leaky gut.

Other factors can also affect the absorption of the nutrients. MTHFR (Methylenetetrahydrofolate Reductase) is one of them (discussed below). Of all the nutrients you need to survive, 90% of them are absorbed in the small intestine. Everything that is not absorbed in the small intestine is then passed onto the large intestine for elimination. I am not a doctor and I do not claim to know the exact names for all the terminology for the digestive process, but I am here to explain it in the simplest terms I can so that you can understand it more fully.

MTHFR: Methylenetetrahydrofolate Reductase is not an organ but we can discuss it here anyway.

I know, it LOOKS like a bad word, but it is not. It is actually a gene mutation that 40- 60% of Americans suffer from. Think about that number a second and how many people that affects. Many people have no idea they have the mutation or have never even heard of it.

The *Genetics Home Reference* offers more detail. This is their definition of the MTHFR gene or Methylenetetrahydrofolate Reductase. "The MTHFR gene provides instructions for making an enzyme called Methylenetetrahydrofolate Reductase. This enzyme plays a role in processing amino acids, the building blocks of proteins. Methylenetetrahydrofolate Reductase is important for a chemical reaction involving forms of the vitamin folate (also called vitamin B9). Specifically, this enzyme converts a molecule called 5,10-Methylenetetrahydrofolate to a molecule called 5-Methyltetrahydrofolate. This reaction is required for the multi-step process that converts the amino acid homocysteine to another amino acid, methionine. The body uses methionine to make proteins and other important compounds."

For the estimated 60 million people affected by this gene mutation--a curse is exactly what it can feel like IF you do not take the right proactive steps. In my language (definition of Rachel) it means that the body cannot take a synthetic nutrient and turn it into a nutrient the body can absorb, or may have a hard time absorbing. So you end up just peeing out all the essential nutrients your body needs.

Unfortunately, without taking proper proactive health measures, those with a MTHFR mutation are directly predisposed to many serious health problems like: heart disease, hypothyroidism, diabetes, cancer, addictive behaviors (alcohol, drugs, and food), severe depression or anxiety, blood clots, dementia, infertility or increased instance of miscarriages, autoimmune diseases, food allergies, and Neural Tube Defects.

If you have this condition, you NEED a methylated vitamin supplement - one that is already converted because your body doesn't necessarily know how to do it.

The Pancreas: The pancreas has two main jobs, the production of insulin and the production of digestive enzymes. The digestive enzymes or juices produced by the pancreas are released into the small intestine which assists in breaking down foods.

The pancreas produces insulin. Insulin is a hormone that regulates blood sugar levels within the body.

The more sugar, refined flours, and coffee we ingest and take into our bodies, the harder the pancreas has to work.

When the pancreas becomes imbalanced then diabetes or hypoglycemia may develop.

The Thyroid: The pancreas and thyroid are both part of the endocrine system. The endocrine system is made of many feedback loops and their various hormones all communicate to one another. This communication helps make changes to the body to try and keep things in balance.

These systems also work in both directions. They influence each other. In the case of sugar, insulin is released by the pancreas to help the cells of the body absorb sugar so that it can be used. The adrenals release cortisol to help sugar get absorbed by the cells of the body. A hypothyroid state leads to a slow absorption of glucose, and a slower breakdown of insulin. Hypothyroid also affects the decrease of the speed at which glucose is absorbed in the gut, a lower glucose to insulin responses and, finally, less glucose in the cells for the body to use.

All of this means less energy to power your cells and brain and more fatigue. To make matters worse, all of this affects the adrenal glands and the hypothalamus-pituitary-adrenal axis (HPA axis). In order to try and fix the problem of not having enough sugar, the adrenal glands release the stress hormone cortisol to increase glucose in the cells.

Hashimoto's patients have some degree of the sugar imbalance described above. If you are thin, it may be hypoglycemia. If you are overweight, it may be insulin resistance or metabolic syndrome. If you feel better after your eat, you are hypoglycemic. If you are tired after you eat, you may have insulin resistance.

All of this creates a vicious cycle that can stop you from getting better. Hashimoto's patients must take blood sugar problems seriously. You will not get better unless you do address your issues seriously. Level your blood sugar and you will help your thyroid; they are connected.

Immune Protectors: The majority of your immune system is located within the digestive tract, so can you see why it is so important to have a healthy gut when it comes to staying healthy. Your digestive track has tissue called lymphatic tissue. This lymphatic tissue is a major part of your immune system. About seventy percent of this gut associated lymph tissue (GALT) is located in the lining of your digestive tract.

There are clumps or nodules of lymph tissue called peyers patches. These peyers patches contain lymphocytes. The job of the lymphocytes is to attach themselves to bacteria to help rid the bacteria from the gut.

Secretory IgA (S IgA) is an antibody found in saliva and the rest of the digestive tract. These antibodies detect foreign invaders like bacteria, antigens, viruses and parasites. How well your digestive system works to break down and eliminate food is affected by many things. Food choices you are making and your emotional health all impact the effectiveness of the secretory antibodies.

The Appendix: The appendix is the organ people sometimes believe has 'no use' and actually it does have a job. After nutrients have been broken down from the food you eat and that food then is passed into the large intestine it meets up with your appendix.

The appendix is a small sac a few inches in length that hangs on the front of the large intestine. Some doctors believe the appendix does not have a real significant use. While other doctors believe that its job is to secrete mucus that can kill toxins that have entered the large intestine.

The appendix also has lymphatic tissue and may play an important part in our immune system and fighting off bacteria.

The Large Intestine: The large intestine is also known as the colon or your bowels. The large intestine is the last five feet of your digestive tract. The large intestine is just like a large holding tank for your waste. This is where the waste stays until you poop it out. I have heard many different numbers from 5 to 30 pounds of poop that can be stored in your large intestine at any given time. Of course the purpose is not to store that much poop, but sometimes you can get 'backed up' and that is where it stays.

The longer the waste stays in the large intestine the more likely your body is to reabsorb some of the toxins that are just sitting there waiting to be released for elimination. You have mucus to protect the lining of the large intestine. As the waste moves through the large intestine water is absorbed back into the body creating a more solid mass of bacteria, yeast, and fungi, also known as poop.

There are good bacteria and bad bacteria that both reside in the intestines. The good and the bad bacteria are both competing to rule over the gut. Your body should have about 80% good bacteria and about 20% bad bacteria. The problem with most people who have health issues is that this ratio is out of balance.

This can happen by making poor food choices, consuming alcohol, prescription medications taken into the body (at times they are necessary), stress, birth control (again sometimes needed), and antibiotics. I am not saying these are all bad or that we should avoid medication when appropriate. I believe these can be used for good, but when overused it can cause the balance of the bacteria in the body to be more like 80% bad and only 20% good.

When out of balance the bad bacteria acts like wild fire in the body and gut, spreading so fast you can lose control of it. Think of these bad bacteria like roots on a rapidly growing tree taking steroids. Those roots can spread out all over the place, creeping into every opening possible and causing havoc on everything in its path. From this spread of bad bacteria, it can result in health issues that are unwanted problems.

Now back to our waste. The waste that is moved through the large intestine, or colon, can move fast or slow. Muscle contractions help to move the waste. Fiber also helps move waste along the path faster.

The large intestine can become stretched out, when this happens; muscle contractions can become less effective. This can turn into lazy or spastic contractions resulting in the waste sitting longer in the intestines. If this happens toxins can be reabsorbed back into the body causing problems physically and emotionally.

The Liver: The liver is the largest organ in the body. The liver is located above the stomach and it is the only organ that when receiving proper nutritional support can regenerate damaged tissue.

The livers job is to detoxify. When the liver is compromised from poor food choices, sugar, stress, alcohol, medications, environmental chemicals, refined flour, coffee, or food chemicals it will store the overload of all the toxins in not only the liver but in the tissues and organs in the rest of the body. When this takes place health issues that can arise may look like allergies, chronic fatigue, skin irritations, digestive problems, waste elimination problems, brain fog, mood swings, hormone imbalances, a low immune system, and more.

The health of your liver has a drastic impact on the health of the rest of your body. Did you know that the liver takes care of over 500 functions in your body? From the way I see it that is a full time job. The liver works like a giant filter for your blood and is one of the main organs that detoxifies your body.

Nutrients in the liver are sent out through the kidneys and then eliminated out the colon. Bile is created in the liver and stored temporarily in the gall bladder. Bile is what gives poop the brownish color, important to know as a trivia fact, right? Bile helps to lubricate, breaks down fats, and helps with nutrient absorption. Fiber helps flush out bile. A diet high in fat and low in fiber can cause the bile to stay longer and toxins can be reabsorbed back into the body.

Another job the liver has is the production of antihistamines to neutralize allergic reactions. When the liver is overworked, overwhelmed and congested with more toxins than it can handle to detoxify, the liver will produce more histamines. These histamines will trigger an allergic response from foods, environment, allergens, and pollutants all around you. Then these can turn into allergies, hay fever, digestive enzyme issues, headaches, skin conditions, depression, irritability, and fatigue.

I have suffered with allergies my whole life and spent many months of the year miserable and congested. This information was so valuable to me because I can now see how it is all related back to gut health.

Hormones like estrogen and testosterone are metabolized by the liver. When the liver is compromised along with a lack of certain vitamins, and low bacteria in the gut, it can result in toxic estrogen by-products. When these by-products are not eliminated by the colon then certain ailments like PMS, bloating, moodiness, and other hormone related issues will arise.

Other hormones that are metabolized in the liver are cortisol and adrenaline. Cortisol is the stress controller, which is the flight or fight hormone. When we live in a life of worry, stress, frustration, and anger these hormones can actually poison us.

Hormones can stay in the liver stored up for about a year. When stored up they cause hormone imbalances and also things like chronic depression or anger can develop. When this happens it also suppresses the immune system and we know how bad that can be when we want to stay healthy.

We should thank our liver every day for helping almost every bodily function run smoothly. We should take care of our precious liver and not abuse it.

Once you understand the body's organs and systems you can start to change things in your health to improve them. Sleep, medication, movement, emotional health, and diet all are things you can do as a starting point when your organs are sending messages (singing to you) that something is not right.

Megan, Canadian mom of six, shares the impact her poor gut health was having on her ability to enjoy life to the fullest.

I am grateful to be able to share a little bit about my story and journey with gut health!

I have been taking gut health supplements for almost 16 months and I have seen some pretty amazing results!

Since the surprise announcement of our sixth child (almost six years ago) I had really been struggling with depression and anxiety. I had not realized the grasp it had taken on my life and the perception I had of myself.

I lived in a cloud of darkness but I still had five other busy kids and a husband I loved, and I needed to show up for them. I put on a smile (the best I could) and I tried to get the essentials done.

That was my new daily goal. Keep everyone alive and well, end of story.

No extras no fluff, if we all got food at least two times a day and they had clothes to wear and I could get them where they needed to be that was enough.

I beat myself up about it.

I depended heavily on my oldest daughter because my husband was traveling all the time. I just could not do the things I used to do to be a fun and happy mom. Everything was a chore, it was hard. There was not a lot of joy.

It got moderately better once my baby was born, at least I was not nauseous and sick twenty-four/seven but my energy levels plummeted. I had no real desire to do anything but sleep!

I figured it was just the newborn phase but when she was three, and then four, I could not really use that as an excuse anymore!

I had a really hard time falling asleep and I had zero energy throughout the day. My IBS was getting worse and I was becoming more and more sensitive to foods I was eating and in turn really struggling with gaining weight.

I decided that enough was enough! This could not be what life was going to be like from now on! I had been watching a few of my friends have such great success with these all natural supplements and they were even creating a financial future for their family sharing them with others!

When I saw that my friend was able to retire her husband who is an ER doctor from two of his other jobs I thought this is exactly what I need! This is the answer to my prayers! Could this be the answer to everything? So I jumped in with both feet!

Within the first week I noticed I had good energy throughout the entire day and that I was not snapping at my kids! I felt more calm and genuinely happy, it was amazing!

I called my husband and told him that he had to start taking all of the same products as me! He has seen some great improvements in his energy, focus and health as well!

I have been able to fall asleep great and wake up feeling rested and ready for the day! My tummy issues are pretty much gone and I have even been regular for the first time in my life! No more cramping and bloating and stomach upset!

The inflammation in my knees is gone and not bothering me at all! But the best thing is that I feel like my old happy self! Megan is back. My depression and anxiety are gone!

I have become passionate about sharing it with others! I am building my own business sharing these supplements with others and building my financial future! I have goals that I never even dreamed about making before coming about!

The idea of one day retiring my husband so that he does not need to travel all the time for work and he can spend time with us and be here with us would be a dream come true! All while getting healthy and feeling the best we have felt in years! It really is so exciting!

Secret 11

Are You Inviting Disease to Your Gut Health Party

Research shows gut bacteria in healthy people is very different than the gut bacteria in people with disease and illness. People who have an illness or disease may lack certain types of bacteria or just have less or too much of a certain type. They may also lack bacteria as a whole. All these factors affect the overall health of the gut microbiome. Certain types of bacteria may keep certain people at a higher risk for developing issues while other types of bacteria prevent them.

I want to share with you my friend Ricci. Her story is nothing short of inspiring! Ricci is an Integrative Nutritional Health Coach and a Guru on all things plant-based and root healing with food. She started her own coaching business, Foodlove By Ricci, where she helps people create healing in every area of their lives. She suffered from debilitating Rheumatoid Arthritis, and traveled the world searching for holistic approaches to healing.

She has created healing for herself through her plant-based diet and the highest quality, appropriate supplementation. She has become an expert on these methods of healing and even appears on the television show Good Things Utah to share her knowledge!

She not only cooks amazing, clean, healthy food but she finds ways to re-create the 'naughty' foods in a plant-based, clean but yummy way. Going from barely walking to seeing her dancing the night away reminds me of those looking for answers and their positive spirits. Ricci shares,

Almost seven years ago my joints started to swell out of nowhere. I had been battling a bad chest infection for months then BAM! Joints started swelling up!

I went to the doctor thinking I had broken my foot. Well turns out it was arthritis. I went from being a marathon runner to feeling like I was under attack and fighting for my life that winter. I pulled out of the feeling of being attacked, but still felt like I was going to die. Spring came and I was left with joint swelling that hopped around my body with no rhyme or reason.

I had my breast implants removed, root canals removed, mercury out of my mouth, flew all over to doctors, paid BIG money for alternative treatments, and still no relief. Doctors only offered me horrible drugs, pain killers and steroids. I have completely changed my diet and never ever quit trying new things and searching!

I have been diagnosed with everything from Candida, Chronic Strep, Rheumatoid Arthritis, EBV (Epstein-Barr virus), C. Pneumoniae infections, Lyme disease, and more. I have dealt with urinary tract infections, swollen joints, sores in my eyes, cystic acne, fatigue, anxiety and general inflammation. I was down with the worst flare-up I had ever had. Knees, wrists, elbows, fingers, toes, shoulders, you name it and it was full of fluid.

I was at rock bottom emotionally, mentally, and physically when I was convinced to try some natural gut health supplements. After two months of detoxing and ups and downs, suddenly my inflammation melted away.

I am five months in and no swelling in my joints!!! I feel alive, my cystic acne is clearing up and I feel like I am

finally healing!! I almost missed this opportunity because of stubbornness.

I finally realized that maybe this was the answer I was praying for and I better not ignore it!! I feel great and have been overjoyed to help others get help too!

Scientists have begun to draw links between the following illnesses and the bacteria in your gut:

Obesity, diabetes, and heart disease are affected by your metabolism. Your metabolism determines how many calories you get from food and what kinds of nutrients you are absorbing. Too much gut bacteria of the wrong kind can turn fiber into fatty acids. This can cause fat deposits in the liver and lead to metabolic syndrome. Metabolic syndrome can lead to diabetes, heart disease and obesity.

Inflammatory bowel diseases including Crohn's disease and ulcerative colitis are developed in people believed to have a lower level of certain anti-inflammatory gut bacteria. It is believed that some bacteria may make your body attack your intestines and set the stages for these diseases.

Colon cancer studies show that people with colon cancer have a different gut microbiome that include higher levels of disease causing bacteria than healthy people without colon cancer.

Anxiety, depression, and autism are all part of the Gut-Brain connection. Your gut is packed with nerve endings that communicate from the brain to the gut. This is sometimes called the 'Gut Brain Axis.'

Studies have been suggested to link the disorders of the central nervous system to the bacteria in your gut. 90% of Serotonin, which is your happy hormone, is produced in the gut, so you can see that if the gut is affected by bacteria it can affect the serotonin as well.

Arthritis, like rheumatoid arthritis, is thought to be linked to people with greater amounts of bacteria that affect inflammation than people without it.

Those with Thyroid disease, Hashimotos and other autoimmune diseases have been shown to have poor gut health.

Emily and her husband Samuel, parents of a son and a daughter, from Wisconsin, all showed great improvements in their health after they realized the impact their gut health had on their bodies. Emily shared her story of their journey,

As a former skeptic on supplements, I said no to them for over eighteen months. I finally decided to try natural gut health supplements in mid-2017. The changes already to my health, wellness and energy have been incredibly remarkable and life changing. But my gut health journey is greater than just my story. My husband has had similarly incredible health and weight loss benefits, and my kids are benefiting from taking gut health supplements too.

The only thing we did differently was start gut health supplements - which had a waterfall effect of eliminating our food cravings and overeating tendencies, and has provided good clean energy that got us both back and passionate about exercise again. But it is more for us than just weight loss. Here is a summary of our amazing journey so far:

Before finding the right gut health supplements for me, I was pretty well read about gut health, as I have been managing my auto-immune disease (Lupus), and not taking any medicine for it through a strict all-natural vegan diet. This was coupled with working to balance my microbiome for years - since the root cause of my disease was stemming in the poor state of my gut health. However, over those years, I went through hundreds of different gut health supplements, different combinations of anti-fungals, and supplements. I wasted a lot of money because nothing worked easily or well, and I was still struggling a bit to find the right balance.

My strictly natural, unprocessed and plant-based vegan diet (with an emphasis on fermented foods) helped, but it was a delicate balance I struggled with constantly.

Then in the two years following the birth of my daughter, and following rounds of IV antibiotics, my body and my gut eventually became completely out of balance, the symptoms of my auto-immune disease were returning, and 'nothing' I did to try to fix it was working. I wasted so much money on inferior supplements and probiotics and felt I was just getting worse.

One night in the beginning of July 2017, I was completely fed up and disgusted with my weight gain, overeating, cravings for (vegan) junk food and late night eating habits that I just could not break. Even worse than that, I was wholeheartedly disappointed by the returned body and joint aches, lethargy, brain fog, water retention, returning skin rashes and other auto-immune related symptoms.

That same night I saw a post on social media about gut health education from my childhood friend, and remembered a trial pack of one of the natural supplements that she sent me back in December 2015. While I trusted my friend and knew she was a smart person, I had been so skeptical of her supplements and ended up just putting that trial pack in the back of my cabinet. I had always read her posts on social media over the course of the year and a half, but just never wanted to try it - AT ALL. After confirming that the old trial pack had not yet expired, the next day I finally gave that seven day pack a try. Over the course of the seven day trial, I noticed changes in my body, in my energy, in the way I was feeling in general and it clicked that there was something in this that might work for me.

I was excited that these products might actually work. I contacted my friend immediately and let her know I finally came around and was ready to give these gut health supplements a real try. I did, and was shocked that my body responded remarkably well - and in a very short time. The impact to my health, wellness and energy has been outstanding. All of my auto-immune symptoms that were returning went away.

My energy was incredible and my mood was up as well. I felt fantastic and was no longer a slave to drinking coffee all day.

In fact, I felt so good that I decided to start running again (after a five plus year hiatus from being a regular runner) which has been amazing. After seeing the positive changes that I was experiencing, my husband wanted in and started the same supplements shortly after I had.

He has had similar fantastic results for weight loss and eliminated cravings as I did - but also found relief for his lactose intolerance and other digestive issues. The biggest shock for him was that his severe seasonal allergies that he struggled with for most of his life never came at him this fall season. He is running again as well and even mixes in swimming and weight lifting regularly now.

His eating habits have also changed: he used to eat a lot of junk food and fast food, and he now food preps with me, choosing lean proteins and veggies, which he enjoys and now craves. We are both rapidly losing weight - to date we have each lost twenty-five pounds and are down multiple clothing sizes. The additional bonding in our relationship over all of it has been another bonus – we have had so much fun in our renewed health and in our journey. It's been exciting!

While the weight loss is great, the internal health benefits are even greater. In July, back when I was feeling my worst and was only a few days into my supplements, I had a full blood work panel done as part of my annual physical and also a testing of ANA counts (auto-immune response markers) that I have scheduled semi-regularly to ensure there are no changes to the status of my Lupus - which had been considered in remission since late 2014. In that July testing, my ANA counts were back, at a moderate level, indicating an auto-immune response was again occurring in my body. My cholesterol was up (although as a vegan, still low), fasting glucose was higher and of course, my weight, and waist circumference increased. After a few months on these supplements, in September 2017 I had my required biometric screening for work, and I had significant changes to my blood work, as compared to the July testing:

> *-Cholesterol went from 138 to 115 (my doctor remarked that was 'in utero' levels that he has never seen before and asked me a lot of detail this time about my plant-based diet),*
> *- Triglycerides went from 89 to 78,*
> *- Fasting glucose went from 94 to 83,*
> *-Waist circumference went down two inches.*

I have not yet had a follow up testing of my ANA counts, but I know my body and I am confident that the auto-immune response is gone again. I will be having them tested again in a few weeks and look forward to it this time.

I have also successfully weaned off of my beta blocker that I had been on since I was twenty-one years old. I had an uncontrollable arrhythmia condition and had a procedure called an RF catheter ablation done to my heart when I was twenty-one. This corrected the arrhythmia, but after wards, my resting heart rate was still very high, so I was put on a low dose of a beta blocker.

I had tried to wean off of the the medication two different times in my life and had uncomfortable side effects, so I always stayed on it. I weaned off of my medication at the end of August and had no issues during the weaning nor after, which is incredible for me personally as I never liked taking medication of any kind.

Similarly, my husband had his annual biometric screening in October 2017. Over his screening from 2016, he also had incredible changes:

- Cholesterol went from 187 to 156
- Triglycerides went from 156 to 116
- Fasting glucose went from 89 to 82
- LDL: went from 119 to 87
-Waist circumference is down three inches.

He had not changed anything about his diet or exercise until right when he started these supplements, which is remarkable.

Our daughter who is two and son, who is five, are also taking probiotics- which their pediatrician enthusiastically approved for them to take. For both, their recurring eczema cleared up within a week or two, and my son, who has suffered with seasonal allergies since he was less than two years old, has not had any allergy symptoms at all this fall so far.

I am so happy with my family's health and wellness improvements, and thankful that I stopped being stubborn and gave them a try. This might sound cliché, but these products have truly changed our lives and our well-being.

We are very consistent with what we take and understand that while our results were rapid, everyone's bodies respond on a different time frame. The key to the weight loss side is that we are not relying on supplements to do the work for us, but rather we feel these supplements are a tool and have found that it is easier to make better choices when our cravings are eliminated and we start wanting healthier *foods. We feel satisfied longer and go through the day without cravings or focusing on what food we can eat next.*

My husband and I both take vitamins, probiotics, and omegas. We absolutely love them and sharing with friends and family has been a multi-faceted added perk in helping others find their journey to a healthier life and lifestyle. These great natural gut health products have been a remarkable blessing in our lives in a short period of time and we look forward to what is in store for us in the future!...

Fast forward a year later and we have both lost just over thirty pounds and have kept it off. Plus, my husband and son's seasonal allergies did not return the following spring or this current fall. My auto-immune disease is still asymptomatic and undetectable in my blood work. It's been amazing!

Secret 12

How Gut Health Makes You Fat or Thin

The average American woman has gone up 20 pounds in weight since the early 1970s. Women are twice as likely as men to have chronic digestive complaints such as Irritable Bowel Syndrome. These complaints usually classified as IBS and the fact that weight is going up are enough to tell us something in our bodies has gone very wrong.

We have known for twenty years that bacteria living in our gut breaks down the food we eat, but we have only recently realized that the microbiome in our gut is not being taken care of properly.

We are wiping out good bacteria by overuse of antibiotics, medication, and other environmental attacks. These attacks can damage the gut bacteria from excessive stress hormones which then cause weight issues, digestive issues, and our immune system to fail.

On the other hand if we can increase this good bacteria and heal our gut, we may be able to change the microbiome enough to have enormous positive effects on how we look and feel.

Talo, father of four, living in Hawaii, shares how he finally made the connection between his weight issues and sweet tooth to his gut. Talo is now healing his body back to better health.

Aloha,

My experience with gut health products have been nothing short of a miracle, at least for me. I now feel good, blessed, and very grateful for the positive health changes I have gained since starting gut health supplements almost 10 months ago.

Prior to adding gut health supplements to my regimen, I was in denial of how bad my health was, I thought I was fine. I was stubborn to listen to my wife for health advice and blind to recognize the red flags that my body was trying to warn me.

The truth is that I already was accepting my current situation as my norm. I was overweight, always tired, my skin was a mess, I had joint pains all over daily, I had gout flares more frequently, sleep deprivation, an uncontrollable sweet tooth and I just was not feeling satisfied or full with the food I ate.

I am happy to say now; all these symptoms have either gone away entirely or are controlled. I enjoy the added energy and how great I feel daily. Supplements for gut health changes lives and I know it can do the same for anyone as it did for me!

Before you eat each day, do you think about what you are putting into your body? Do you think about the foods you eat? Are they processed or are they whole? Are they healthy or are they something that should be avoided?

Most people eat food without really thinking about it. They may think, 'will this taste good?' 'Will this satisfy my craving?' But they do not think twice about what the nutritional value really is.

We know we 'should' eat healthy but we eat what we 'want.' We have been taught since we were kids that we need to eat to survive.

We are a society of instant gratification. We think if we do not eat we will die!

We want something that is quick and easy. We are tired and stressed out and so thinking about driving to a store, shopping, and preparing a meal may seem overwhelming. So we turn to fast food. Fast food eating is at an all-time high. Poor education of eating habits can be partly to blame.

It is not your fault, no one educates on what is really in the food you eat and you are feeding your family. But at some point you need to take responsibility for the food choices and eating habits you have created.

Fast food restaurants feed 50 million customers a day in America. We think bigger is better. The lack of portion control is not addressed until a health issue arises, or a doctor does blood work, or a health scare opens the eyes of the consumer.

We have good intentions but not good follow through.

The fact that the fast food numbers keep going up tells us that we still have a long way to go. Fast food chains are hopping on the bandwagon and offering 'healthier choices,' but you should still be aware of how the food choices affect you.

If we learn more about what we are eating, where it comes from and where it goes, this will help us move forward into a new era where we care more about how our food affects our gut than how it tastes. The habits we are creating are having long term effects on our health, so we need to realize what we do now sets the course for our future.

How much healthier could we be if we started caring now about our food choices and knowing that what we put into our gut will determine the health of our microbiome. When we eat better our gut, which is our second brain, will be much happier and will help our mood, energy levels, and overall happiness in life.

124

Jessica B. A mother of three young kids with a degree in Sociology and Psychology shares,

I want to share my experience with researching and using gut health products because they have made such a impact in my life.

A couple years back, I was suffering from IBS with lots of bloating and gas. I knew all the bathrooms along the freeway and my usual routes... just in case. I was embarrassed to go out with friends just in case I had an episode hit.

I was missing sleep and along with other things I had hypoglycemia too. I was hungry all the time and shaky. I was tired and unhappy. I was trying lots of over the counter medicines along with some herbal stuff. I changed some of the food I ate and nothing was helping. This was not how I was wanting to live my life. I was only in my thirties.

I had a friend of mine that had been given some gut health products from her family and suggested I take some. I had nothing to lose. She gave me a bottle of a magnesium supplement. It sadly sat on my shelf for a few months before I tried it because I was worried I would be stuck on the toilet for a week and I did not have time for that. I am a busy mom of three and wife. I also have a job in a school where you can only take breaks at certain times.

Months later, I was at the city's Fourth of July carnival and ran into an old friend. I worked for her many years back and had not seen her for some time. She was at a booth and I stopped to visit with her. I was wondering about the bottle of magnesium on my shelf and we started talking about gut health and the benefits of supplements.

She had answers! She explained more information about the importance of gut health. I was sold! I started taking the magnesium supplement that had been sitting on my shelf and quickly noticed a change in my stomach.

I slowly added in a probiotic and vitamins to my routine. I was sleeping better, had less shaking and sugar cravings. I did not have to eat all the time. My IBS and bloating decreased a ton. I was getting my life back! I have now tried more gut health products because I know they work! I love learning more about gut health and get excited to share with everyone that I am a Gut Heath Geek now.

Secret 13

What Probiotics Do for You

Prebiotics

Wait, didn't I say I was going to talk about probiotics? Probiotics are a common term that most people have heard before and we will discuss them, but let us start out by going over prebiotics.

Prebiotics are a fiber that feed probiotics. Learning and understanding that prebiotics can feed probiotics is important in helping probiotics flourish in a healthy way. Prebiotics can feed many forms of bacteria. There are some prebiotics that feed all forms of bacteria and there are some prebiotics that feed only certain strains of bacteria. When taking prebiotics it is important to know which strains of bacteria you are feeding.

Prebiotic fiber can come in supplement form and food. Foods that contain prebiotic ingredients, which are mostly fiber, feed the bacteria in the gut producing fermentation by-products that benefit the health. Some prebiotic foods include:

- Almonds
- Asparagus
- Bananas
- Burdock root
- Cereal grains (whole wheat, barley, rye)
- Chicory root
- Endive
- Garlic
- Greens (especially dandelion greens)

- Jerusalem artichoke
- Jicama
- Kiwi
- Leeks
- Legumes
- Mushrooms
- Oats
- Onions
- Salsify (an edible European plant of the daisy family, with a long root like that of a parsnip)

After waking up one day with a frozen shoulder and hip, Deirdre turned her attention to gut health. Now Deirdre, a New York based Entrepreneur, specializes in helping others understand wellness from the Gut-Brain connection.

My gut health journey started over a year ago with a Naturopath. Around when I turned 50, I had some extra stress (kids and elderly parents) and pretty much woke up one day with a frozen shoulder, a frozen hip (did not even know that was a thing), and a stiff neck among other things.

It turns out I had a serious yeast buildup in my brain and at the sites of old injuries from a car accident. I was also bloated and had a lot of cortisol. We worked on my gut health for close to a year. I took tons of supplements, muscle tested every couple of weeks and I significantly improved.

When I learned about a line of supplements that concentrated on mental health, I was intrigued. It was so consistent with everything I had been doing... and a lot cheaper than buying all my supplements a la carte. I was also intrigued because of the mental wellness component since I have had sleep issues most of my life, as well as some issues with mood and anxiety. So when I learned that these supplements contained a package with a combination of strains of probiotics, prebiotics and that have been shown to improve mental wellness I decided to give it a try.

I have noticed that my stress resiliency and sleep have improved significantly. I have had a few dips, but they are short lived and I bounce back quickly. I find it so interesting how specific strains of probiotics work for different things. A year ago my most noticeable issues were physical. Once those resolved, I went deeper and worked on underlying mental wellness issues that I have struggled with for years.

When you eat foods containing prebiotics you are feeding bacteria. Prebiotics do not replace probiotics, they actually work together.

Now think of foods you eat daily, how many contain beneficial prebiotics?

Foods are eaten for many different reasons. Fuel, energy, health, and nutrition are all great reasons to eat. Social, addiction, or even trends are some reasons we consume food in an unhealthy way.

Think about holiday advertising for certain items. St. Patrick's Day shakes, Valentines chocolates, or even a limited time rainbow unicorn sprinkled 1200 calorie 50 grams of sugar specialty drink. If it is advertised 'for a limited time only,' how many people will rush out and go try it just to say 'yeah, I tried it,' knowing it was not good for their health.

They know it is unhealthy, but that does not stop them. If others are trying it, it must be OK! They do not want to 'miss out' so they indulge. Some people eat for the enjoyment and others may eat for the calming effect.

What makes a food calming? Sometimes I think 'everything is calming,' when I eat food I calm down and feel better. But what about eating for emotional reasons? When you eat for emotional reasons you are using food for a quick fix or temporary 'get-away' from a deeper problem. This emotional eating can be very addictive and harmful.

You may have a temporary calming effect, or numbness from the food, but more often than not, it also leaves you with a feeling of guilt. Guilt from eating the item, eating too many calories, eating that leads to more weight gain, more sugar problems, and more stress. These are not calming foods in a healthy way.

Stressful events in your life that are big or small can cause cortisol levels to rise in your body. Raised cortisol causes food cravings. In women those cravings tend to be the strongest for carbohydrates, especially sweet foods.

The more carbohydrates and sugars you eat make your mood get worse and your stress level higher. You become part of this vicious cycle of stress that leads to high cortisol, high cortisol that leads to food cravings, and poor food choices that causes stress to go higher.

Not fair? Well there is more. High cortisol also triggers an enzyme in our fat cells. This enzyme converts cortisol to more cortisol. The fat cells called visceral, which are the ones over our abdomen protecting our vital organs, have more of these enzymes than the subcutaneous fat cells, which are in our butt and thighs. This is why woman under stress tend to accumulate more belly fat.

I looked at this as an 'aha moment' where it all made sense. I struggled with fat cells in my abdomen my whole life and learning about the relation to poor gut health, and high cortisol helped me pull it all into place of why I struggled. Now I know that if I am working on gut health, which helps blood sugar regulate and cortisol be in normal levels, I am at the same time helping those fat cells not expand. Win, Win, for me and everyone else that has been struggling with their growing waist.

When I talk about real calming foods, I do not mean emotional temporary support foods. I mean meals and snacks that will truly soothe and calm you. It may be because of the specific nutrients the calming foods provide or the steady reliable source of energy they give you, but these are foods that really benefit your body. These foods can help you feel focused and balanced and help you accomplish anything.

Foods that have a calming effect can help to fight stress, which then helps prevent gut health issues and those unwanted cortisol issues. These calming foods are different from comfort foods you may eat when emotionally stressed. When you are tired and drained you choose foods that mostly contain sugar and carbohydrates. The right kind of calming foods can help you feel better and stay calmer. Some great calming foods are:

Asparagus

This vegetable is very high in folate which may help to keep your cool. The only drawback from these slender delicious treasures is that they may make your urine smell funny. As long as you are not taking people to the bathroom with you, you should be fine.

Avocados

Rich in glutathione, these creamy fruits are a great stress-relief on your body. Glutathione is a substance that blocks intestinal absorption of certain fats. Avocados also contain lutein, beta-carotene, vitamin E, vitamin B and more folate than any other fruit. Avocados can be counted as a fat so just use portion control when eating this yummy fruit. They are a great addition in smoothies.

Berries

Blueberries have some of the highest levels of an antioxidant known as anthocyanin. Anthocyanin has been linked to all kinds of positive health outcomes, including sharpened thinking. All berries including strawberries, raspberries and blackberries are rich in vitamin C. Vitamin C has been shown to help reduce stress levels. Some people have been given vitamin C to help lower blood pressure and cortisol. Berries are a great menu item all the time.

Cashews

A great source of protein and with portion control they are a great snack. I love nuts and I could eat them all the time. For those trying to lose weight they are a great combination of protein and fat. Cashews are also a great source of zinc. People with depression and anxiety have reported lower levels of zinc. Since our bodies have no way of storing zinc it is important to get some every day in our diet.

Chamomile Tea

These pretty little flowers have a great bedtime soothing effect. Just pour a cup of boiling water over 2 to 3 heaping tablespoons of the dried flowers (you can buy chamomile either loose or in tea bags at health food stores) and steep for 10 minutes. It is a great way to finish the day. A study from the University of Pennsylvania tested chamomile supplements on 57 participants with generalized anxiety disorder for 8 weeks, and found it led to a significant drop in anxiety symptoms. And yes, according to the University of Maryland Medical Center, there is some evidence that, in addition to calming nerves, chamomile promotes sleep.

Chocolate

One of my favorites, but besides the healthy antioxidants in this treat, it also has an undeniable link to mood. A recent study from the University of California, San Diego, School of Medicine reports that both women and men eat more chocolate as depressive symptoms increase. So that is evidence that chocolate does make you feel better. Dark chocolate, in particular, is known to lower blood pressure, which then helps you in feeling calm. It contains more polyphenols and flavonols (two important types of antioxidants) than most fruit juices. You can stay on track with your weight loss goals even with an occasional snack of dark chocolate once a week. I love the European chocolate the best.

Garlic

Garlic contains allicin, which has been linked to help prevent heart disease, cancer, and even the common cold (thank you garlic!) Garlic is packed with powerful antioxidants. Antioxidants neutralize free radicals. Free radicals are particles that damage our cells, cause diseases, and encourage aging. Antioxidants also reduce and help prevent some of the damage the free radicals cause over time. We need garlic in our lives when stress comes into play, which can be all the time for some of us. Stress weakens the immune system and garlic can help bring it back up. Garlic is great added to many dishes; just watch out for too much in your food or it may cause garlic breath.

Grass-fed Beef

Grass-fed beef has more antioxidants, vitamin C, vitamin E and beta-carotene than grain-fed beef. Grass-fed beef does not have added hormones, antibiotics, or other drugs.

Grass-fed beef is healthier to eat. It is also lower in fat overall and has four times the omega 3's. A study in the *British Journal of Nutrition* found that healthy volunteers who ate grass-fed meat increased their blood levels of omega-3 fatty acids and decreased their levels of pro-inflammatory omega-6 fatty acids. These changes have been linked with a lower risk of disorders, including cancer, cardiovascular disease, depression, and inflammatory diseases. Grass-fed beef is pricey but well worth the occasional splurge.

Oatmeal

Talk about a favorite comfort food! A complex carbohydrate, oatmeal causes your brain to produce serotonin, a feel-good chemical. Not only does serotonin have antioxidant properties, it also creates a soothing feeling that helps overcome stress. Studies have shown that kids who eat oatmeal for breakfast stay sharper throughout the morning.

Beta-glucan, the type of soluble fiber found in oatmeal, has been shown to promote greater satiety scores than other whole grains. Make a batch of the steel-cut variety on the weekend, store it in the fridge, and microwave it on busy mornings. It keeps beautifully, and in fact, that is how restaurants often prepare it. I start a batch at night in the Crockpot and it is ready for early morning breakfast. I love to add sliced apples, chia seeds and walnuts to my breakfast delight.

Oranges

A vitamin C powerhouse, oranges have the added benefit of being totally portable. That tough skin keeps them protected while they are bouncing around in your purse or backpack, you can tote them anywhere. Experiment with all the varieties like clementines, tangelos, and mineola's. The more I eat them the more I love them. The easy to peal cuties are a favorite with my kids.

Oysters

Some people believe oysters are only good as aphrodisiacs! They belong here, as well, because they are the king of zinc. Six oysters, which are what you would typically be served in a restaurant as an appetizer, have more than half the RDA for this important mineral.

Walnuts

The sweet flavor of walnuts is so pleasant, and it is nice to know they have been proven to provide a bit of a cognitive edge. They contain alpha-linolenic acid, an essential omega-3 fatty acid, and other polyphenols that have been shown to help prevent memory loss. To keep them fresh I store mine in the freezer. I love to chop them up and add them to salads, yogurts, and breads.

When anxiety from poor gut health becomes crippling it can make even a small errand or task feel impossible to accomplish. Shalamar a swimming instructor and mom of three, shares how the use of probiotics and vitamins has helped her accomplish responsibilities of motherhood even better.

Being out in public may seem like no big deal to most people.

Most people can run their errands, go out with friends, attend social gatherings, enjoy family activities or go grocery shopping like it is just another day. For someone with social anxiety, these tasks feel like diving deep underwater, then swimming back up to the surface, only to find the surface is farther away than it seems so you suddenly feel as if you are about to drown.

For years, I have had to take medication right before I would leave my house, just so I could function like a normal human being. It was crippling! As I've started my gut healing journey with probiotics, prebiotics, and vitamins, my anxiety has lessened very slowly. I still have really bad days, don't get me wrong. But!! I'm having more and more good days.

Days where I can leave my house and still be able to breathe. Days when I can be out in public and enjoy my kids instead of being irritated, short of breath, and scared they are going to be kidnapped. Days when I can see the beauty in the commotion of society.

THIS is why I continue to talk about gut health. THIS is why I reach out to EVERYONE.

The other day I was able to take my kids to the dentist. After the dentist I took them to McDonald's because they did not have any cavities. This is a big treat for them. We live in a small town where the only fast food restaurant is Subway. Then we met my husband and went to the movie theater. I was able to enjoy my day without being medicated. I felt calm and was able to focus.

THIS is a huge victory for me.

A few months ago, I remember asking my mom if people's faces change as they get older because I felt like I looked different but could not figure out why. I was scrolling through my pictures and was pretty shocked to see what I looked like at the beginning of the year. Then I realized it was the puffiness in my face?! That is inflammation! After I started to heal my gut, I keep noticing small changes in my body that I was not expecting. I never realized how much inflammation I had internally until it was gone! I just thought, 'this is me. I have a big, round, chubby face.'

Gut health and anti-inflammatory supplements along with probiotics and prebiotics have helped decrease inflammation in my body and I can feel it. I just never thought I would see the effects on the outside!

Guys, I love my products! The longer I've been on them, the better I feel mentally, emotionally, and physically!

The longer I take them, the more I realize how life changing healing your gut can be.

Probiotics

Now we can get to Probiotics.

The health of your gut is extremely important to your overall well-being. Your gut is responsible for the important functions of the body's digestive and immune systems. Beneficial bacteria in your gut have the capability of affecting so many functions in your body. Your body's ability to absorb vitamins, how your immune system responds, the regulation of hormones, proper digestion, produce vitamins, the ability for the body to eliminate toxins, and your overall mental health are all affected by the health of the gut and the amount of beneficial bacteria residing there. The overall variety of your gut flora is vitally essential to your overall well-being. This is the reason probiotics are necessary to restoring your gut health to a more balanced and normal state. The probiotics help to re-populate all that good bacteria in the gut and the varieties needed for a flourishing microbiome.

When shopping around to buy a probiotic it is important to note that most probiotics differ in both their bacterial composition and quality. There are hundreds of commercially available probiotic supplements to choose from. Many of these are single strains. Others contain multiple strains. The concentration of bacteria in each strain in the probiotics can vary as well.

This is important to remember when choosing a probiotic because there are many probiotics that claim to help, when in reality, they do not have enough bacteria to alter the gut flora it may promise to help. Some probiotics have a good amount of bacteria, and multiple strains, but do not survive long enough to reach the gut and therefore do not help at all.

Your gut needs a lot of tender loving care, how you treat it, and what you put in it will determine your body's ability to thrive in a healthy way. I was someone who took probiotics for over 25 years before I found one that I could tell was making a difference. If you are struggling to find a good probiotic that will make a difference reach out and I will share with you the ones I found that made a difference in my health.

Probiotics are key to introducing good bacteria into your system which will restore and replenish your gut flora. Restoring the gut flora will result in improving the quality of your life and long-term prevention of gut related issues.

Many foods contain probiotics. I call these foods probiotic power foods.

Probiotic power foods are amazing foods that are good for your gut. Some of those probiotic foods are fermented foods. Fermented foods like Kombucha are all the 'buzz' these days. You can find aisles of Kambucha drinks in many grocery store aisles. Probiotic fermented foods start as whole foods and with the help of microorganisms, the sugars and carbohydrates in them are converted to compounds like lactic acid. Lactic acid is what gives pickles and sauerkraut their sour taste. When you drink Kombucha it has a sort of 'kick' to it that is the lactic acid. Instead of being cooked or eaten fresh, these power foods filled with probiotics are prepared by putting them in a slow cooker or a mason jar. This allows the bacteria to ferment them naturally.

Bacteria, like lactobacilli, break down the sugars into acids, preserving the food and producing a salty and tangy flavor. Fermented foods can also provide prebiotic fiber for your gut bacteria. You get a 2 for 1 combo with fermented foods in that they have prebiotics and probiotics in one source.

These boosted levels of probiotic foods can increase the level of good bacteria in your gut or digestive tract. By doing this you will improve health and balance your body's microbiome to a healthier level. Fermented foods are easier to digest in your stomach and break down because the digestive process has already begun.

Some of the fermented foods that might actually taste pretty good include:

Fermented Beverages: Kombuchas and Kvass.

Kombucha is a naturally effervescent tea created by combining black tea, natural sugars, bacteria and yeast. The bacteria and yeast consume the sugar, producing a fizzy, tangy drink high in probiotics, B vitamins, and acetic acid, which studies have shown can help stabilize blood glucose levels and boost satiety. Kombucha can come in may fruity flavors, making it easier and tastier to drink.

Kvass is an Eastern European fermented drink produced similarly to kombucha, but traditionally made with rye bread and various veggies as opposed to tea. Currently the process to make it often skips the bread and is made with just veggies and fruit, a bit of salt, and bacteria and yeast. This results in a fizzy, tangy, and sometimes a bit salty beverage. All varieties contain probiotics, but the health benefits will vary depending on the produce used.

Fermented Dairy: Yogurt, kefir, buttermilk, and some cheeses.

Yogurts labeled with the phrase, 'contains live and active cultures' guarantees to have 100 million probiotic cultures per gram in a cup of yogurt. You do have to be careful of yogurts with a lot of sugar in them. The sugar might be counteracting the good bacteria you are putting into your gut by feeding the bad bacteria.

Kefir, another fermented milk product, tastes like a slightly tangier, yet drinkable yogurt and boasts even more probiotics. Both are also good sources of protein, calcium, and vitamin D.

Cultured Non-Dairy Products: Yogurts and kefirs made from organic soy, coconut, etc.

Cultured coconut milk yogurt is great if you cannot or do not want to have dairy in your diet. A cultured coconut milk, found in coconut milk yogurt, is made by adding various live active cultures to the coconut milk and fermenting until it is loaded with probiotics.

Fermented Soybeans: Tempeh and miso.

Tempeh, is a cousin of tofu but has a nuttier taste. Tempeh is made from soybeans that have been fermented with a fungus starter. It is loaded with iron, potassium, magnesium, calcium, and protein. Like tofu, it contains all essential amino acids, so it is a complete source of vegetarian protein. It is also easier to digest than other soy-based products because it is fermented,. This versatile superfood works great in stir-fry and even as a meat replacement in burgers.

Miso a Japanese seasoning, is made from fermenting soybeans with salt, a fungus starter, and sometimes grains such as barley or brown rice. It is sold as a paste that can be added to soups, stir-fry, and smoothies.

Fermented Vegetables: Kimchi, sauerkraut, carrots, green beans, beets, lacto-fermented pickles, and traditional cured Greek olives.

The fermented vegetables which are preserved with a natural lacto-fermentation, as opposed to being brined in vinegar, are highest in probiotics. These include sauerkraut and kimchi (both made from vitamin C and fiber rich cabbage), and traditional sour or dill pickles. Pasteurized versions of these products, which include most mainstream brands, do not contain probiotics because they are heated to a temperature that destroys all good and bad bacteria. To ensure you are getting the real deal, look for terms on the label like 'unpasteurized,' 'naturally fermented,' 'raw,' or 'contains live and active cultures.' Of course, as with any unpasteurized food, your risk for food borne illness is a bit greater, so be sure to refrigerate these products after opening and consume them by the date on the label.

Fermented Grains and Beans: Lacto-fermented lentils, chickpeas, etc.

As with the vegetables make sure the grains and beans have not been pasteurized. Look for the same terms on the labels like 'unpasteurized,' 'naturally fermented,' 'raw,' or 'contains live and active cultures.

Fermented Condiments: Raw apple cider vinegar, etc.

Yep, now you can even buy probiotic-boosted ketchup, thanks to the emerging trend of fermented condiments.

Katie, mom of five and military wife from Georgia, shares how she struggled like a lot of moms do after having children.

Before I started to work on my gut health I had my 3rd baby. I had Postpartum Depression (PPD) that stemmed from the baby having colic and basically being alone right after having a baby. I had moved to a new state, with no friends and no one wanting to even try to get to know me.

That PPD turned into full-blown depression and anxiety. I never took my kids out, I was always tired, I did not have the energy to take my kids anywhere, we always stayed at home, and I never did activities with my kids, heck I would not even read to them most days! It was horrible! My husband and I fought almost daily, and the fights just got worse every day, my kids ignored me and I was severely overwhelmed by my life.

Within a month of starting some new supplements to help heal my gut my husband noticed a difference with me. He knew the days that I took the products and the days I forgot. We fought less, I was not nearly as tired, I was laughing more again. I wanted to work out. I was an actual mom to my kids again. We read books, run, play, make forts, camp (indoors of course hahaha), bake, and I teach them to cook. I am even getting ready to home-school them which the idea of that would have freaked me out and overwhelmed me before.

I laugh so much more now, I have more patience, I am more willing to look at the good and find the silver lining in all the crazy around me.

My life has not changed, my perspective has.

I can finally be the mom and wife I always wanted to be. I can take my kids in public by myself and not feel anxious that I am going to forget one or lose one (I have 5, with a couple of runners, so it is a legit concern for me). I can even make plans and not back out of them. I can make friends again and not feel like everyone is out to get me or hates me. I can be my fun, loving, kind, outgoing self again and I love it!!!

Saccharomyces Boulardii Fungi or S. Boulardii Fungi

If you are finally experiencing good gut health then congratulations! If you still have some distress signals coming from your body pleading for help, you may need to add in a good fungi. A good source of probiotics may not be enough to have a great flora in your gut garden.

Adding in fungi that can spread and grow may be the answer you are looking for. S. boulardii is a great fungus to add. S. boulardii is yeast, which is a type of fungus so you are good in that department. The hardest part of adding in these fungi is that you may not be able to get enough from whole food that you eat. S. boulardii is in some plants like lychee and mango's (which are delicious), but you would have to eat a lot to reap any of the benefits.

You can get S. boulardii in a supplement form. There are some great supplements that have bacteria, fungi, and digestive enzymes in them. An all in one capsule is an added benefit rather than having to buy everything separate. I can share one I recommend, but you can find it in other options as well.

S. boulardii was previously identified as a unique species of yeast. Now it is believed to be a strain of Saccharomyces cerevisiae (baker's yeast).

S. boulardii is also used as medicine. S. boulardii is most commonly used for treating and preventing diarrhea, including rotaviral diarrhea in children, diarrhea caused by an overgrowth of "bad" bacteria in adults, traveler's diarrhea, and diarrhea associated with tube feedings. It is also used to prevent and treat diarrhea caused by the use of antibiotics. It may also be used to help with acne.

Remember when adding anything to your health regimen please do your own research and check with your health professional to make sure you are educated and understand how to incorporate it in your lifestyle and if something new is right for you.

Abygale, homeschooling mom of three, from Missouri, shares how the healing process of the gut is an ongoing journey, not a destination.

My friend and I were on a road trip to visit my dad for spring break. I remember stopping at a gas station and getting the phone call that would change my life, but not in the way you think. My dad said he and my step-mom would not be home when we got there because my step-brother was having heart issues and they were rushing to Oklahoma City to be with him.

From that phone call on, anxiety had entered my life. I felt panic. My heart was racing. I was already a little nervous making a long road trip in a car I had been driving less than a week. I returned from that trip and went to see my nurse practitioner. She prescribed a medication that would make me drowsy and therefore, less anxious. I hated being drowsy all the time. It was either that or moderate to severe anxiety constantly.

I was working full time and going to college full time and that was hard all by itself. I went through several other medications over the years. None made me feel even keel without weird side effects. During those years, I also began suffering from depression on and off. I knew there had to be different answers, but I just did not have the right tools to find the information I needed.

Three years ago, I started hearing things here and there about the Gut-Brain connection. As the months passed and the studies grew more abundant, I learned that depression and anxiety are mostly problems that come from poor gut health. I had tried some inferior probiotics in the past, but they did not bring the results I was hoping.

About a year ago, I began taking gut health supplements, including a superior probiotic that have changed my life. I am not where I want to be yet, but that is ok. I know gut healing takes time. The gut health supplements have helped me to have significantly less anxious feelings and less down days. I also have better sleep, mood, confidence, outlook on life, less sickness, and more energy to be a mom, wife, home-school teacher, and business owner.

Now, I have found a better way. I do not have to feel numb or drowsy. Being able to be who I truly am is one of the greatest gifts I have received.

Secret 14

Only You Can Make a Change

Take a Stand

The average American wants gratification now with consequences later. If they knew all the secrets to gut health they could start making changes now and not wait until it is too late.

You must learn to take a stand for your health, become educated, and improve your gut health before it controls you. No one can do it for you, you have to decide and then take action for yourself.

So what can you do now to take that stand? Through testing, nutritional changes, supplements, and sometimes even mindset, it is possible to reverse and repair the damage that has been done to your gut over years of unhealthy diets or imbalances. It is never too late to improve your health.

Given the proper tools your body has the ability to heal itself. You may just need a little help to get started. Let's recap what we have talked about so far.

To start you need to figure out what is really going on inside your body. With advanced diagnosis testing to determine what food sensitivities you may have that could be affecting your body's ability to absorb nutrients or digest, you will have a starting point.

Make a plan that has attainable goals. Do not think you are going to heal your gut in 30 days and be able to go back to the lifestyle you had before. It will take some time. You may need to meet with a certified nutrition expert to start a nutrition plan that matches your lifestyle complemented with ongoing counseling. Find an expert that really understands gut health and is willing to work with you to improve it.

A good regimen will work on removing problem foods and toxins from your body that could be causing the issues. A good regimen will also work on restoring the nutrients your body is lacking. Think detox and replenish, detox and replenish, detox and replenish. When gut healing has begun and you are on a clean diet with proper supplementation including probiotics, you will start to restore and get closer to an ideal balance of good gut bacteria. You can then maintain your optimal levels and continue to support and promote a healthy digestive tract. Remember the line 'You are what you eat' that will start to mean more to you every day.

Because of all this modern day 'food science,' we are actually deficient in a lot of basic nutrients and that contributes to so many illnesses. Even those of us who live relatively healthy lifestyles can lack in energy and struggle to lose weight. We have nutrients that are not getting absorbed into the body properly. Maybe they are synthetic and your body is lacking the ability to absorb them, or maybe there are just not enough nutrients in our depleted soil where foods are grown. The fact is that we cannot receive all the nutrients we need by diet alone. Supplementation is absolutely needed for proper gut health.

Supplements can help your body receive the proper nutrients it is lacking. We do not eat a perfect diet on a daily basis. We eat foods that have traveled from far distances and are picked before they are ripe. We eat foods that have been processed or have chemicals, toxins, pesticides, or unnatural additives in them. Supplements can include added in methylated vitamins, minerals, probiotics, prebiotics, and enzymes.

Methylated supplements give your body a much better chance of absorbing the nutrients instead of just peeing all the good nutrients out. Researching supplements that could benefit your gut to stay as healthy as possible will benefit you for years to come.

Probiotics and prebiotics can help to increase the good bacteria needed in your microbiome, but you need to get a good variety, one strain alone will not do it. You need to work on killing off the bad bacteria, so that the good bacteria can thrive. Our bodies will always have a small ratio of bad bacteria. It is when that bad bacteria gets out of control that we need to be concerned. So, if you constantly work on killing excess bacteria you can help that balance stay at a healthy ratio.

Probiotics prevent the adhesion of pathogenic bacteria of the intestine, help to heal leaky gut and restore gut integrity by improving the good bacteria to a healthy balance. Once a healthy balance is obtained using probiotics in a synergistic combination with prebiotics to maintain gut health it will help prevent gut issues from coming back.

Enzymes are a great addition to the diet. Digestive enzymes can help to break down processed food. Whole foods are full of digestive enzymes but foods that have been processed are lacking enzymes entirely. In a gut full of western diet processed foods the gut needs to have a way to be able to break down the processed foods to digest them properly. If the body is not getting the enzymes it needs from the foods eaten the body will try to pull them from other sources. This leaves a deficiency somewhere else in the body.

Enzymes are also used to break down certain types of bad bacteria. Enzymes have several different purposes that are all useful in the health of the gut.

Current western medical research is much more focused on the treatment of disease rather than focusing on the prevention of disease. The treatment of disease is just a Band-Aid for health and is not solving the issues at hand. I believe that as time goes on we will see more and more people wanting to increase their knowledge on gut health to get to the root of the issues they are having. They will want to treat the problem not just cover it up with a Band-Aid. More people will want to increase their gut health to prevent health issues later in life.

More people will care about their bodies.

You can eat a nutritious diet high in fiber like fruits, vegetables, whole grains, and a minimal consumption of red meat.

Remember a diet high in fat and sugar and low in fiber can kill certain types of gut bacteria, making your microbiome less diverse in a variety of good bacteria.

Exercise can also encourage the growth of a variety of gut bacteria. Having a variety of good gut bacteria promotes better health and in return reduces your risk of disease. If you have never exercised, or if it has been a while, start small. Incorporate 15-20 minutes of moving and go up from there as your body gets physiological benefits from exercising.

Park your car far away and take the stairs instead of the elevator. Invite your family to take a walk after dinner. Join a gym with friends, or meet at the park and workout while your kids play. Find what you love to do and make it enjoyable. Then as you feel better and get stronger increase that time until you are doing a full workout. Life is to be enjoyed not just endured.

Tobacco abstinence, alcohol abstinence, maintenance of normal body weight, avoidance of non-steroidal anti-inflammatory drug (NSAID) ingestion and control of your stress can support gut health.

Meditative methods that often originate from traditional Chinese medicine and other Asiatic cultures (for example, Ayurveda and Tai-Chi) are growing popularity and becoming increasingly accepted by health professionals as valuable tools to maintain gut health and general well-being. Relax and breathe for 10 minutes a day, clear your mind and feel better.

Stay away from antibiotics and other medications that destroy the good bacteria. Sometimes medication may be necessary to take. Western medicine tends to prescribe antibiotics and medication way too often without looking at the effects these medications have on the long-term health of our gut.

Cherstyn, mom of 6 from Utah, and a Director of Development for a nonprofit charity, shares how she broke down her health testimony into several 'pockets' or parts to see how it all fits together.

My Health Part 1: Migraines

For a while now I have considered breaking down my health issues from the start, showing how they built upon each other, and how I came to learn all that I know today about true, long-term healing from the inside out.

In seventh grade I woke up one morning with strange vision obstructions, my right hand was tingling, and I was unable to grasp any objects. I had slurred speech. These symptoms were similar to a stroke and then horrible head pain kicked in.

As a seventh grader I had a neurologist who diagnosed me with severe, complicated migraines. As if common migraines were not bad enough, I had complicated migraines which mimicked stroke symptoms.

I began my first bottle of prescriptions at that young age to manage the pain. I had 3 to 5 migraines a week sometimes. This went on, with fluctuating degrees of intensity, for 20 years.

Today there are countless studies on the connection between gastrointestinal health and migraine headaches. Research finds that higher prevalence of headaches go hand-in-hand with those who regularly experience negative G.I. symptoms.

I also had been colicky as a baby, and research suggests that colic is an early life expression of migraines, again, linked to gut health.

So there is part one of my health journey... I had no idea that my migraines had anything at all to do with my next health issue....

My Health Part 2: *Painful Periods, Cystic Acne, Sugar Cravings*

In part 1 I discussed the start of my migraine headaches in junior high and how that was a very early sign of poor gut health.

Part 2 introduces my next indicators of that same root cause... painful periods, cystic acne, and intense sugar cravings.

A lot of girls can relate to painful periods, needing a heating pad and curling up in a ball on your bed after taking high doses of ibuprofen. It usually lasted through the first day, maybe into the second day with most girls, and then they could breathe a sigh of relief until next month.

Mine were a bit worse than that. I had all of the above symptoms, but I also would get a fever, was nauseous, and had to have a prescription for the pain because ibuprofen would not touch it. I went to an OB/GYN for the prescription. So now I had a neurologist for my migraines and an OB/GYN for my painful periods.

Around this time I also began to get acne; deep cystic acne that was very tender to the touch and of course unsightly.

I found a dermatologist, and yet again another prescription. At the time it was antibiotics, and little did I know that antibiotics would only exacerbate the problem in my gut even further.

This is a good time to mention sugar cravings. A lot of kids have a sweet tooth, and I certainly did. Some people claim that sugar caused acne, and others claimed it was unrelated. I was a healthy person in many ways, and chose a healthy diet, but I always had to have dessert. Daily.

A compromised gut leads to inflammation, and inflammation in the gut causes inflammation elsewhere like acne, painful periods, weight gain, sugar cravings, bloating, and even my future endometriosis. That is just to name a few; there is much much more.

Sugar cravings and consumption negatively affect the menstrual cycle because blood sugar levels need to be balanced in order to have healthy hormone function.

Caffeine, stress, antibiotics, prescriptions, birth control, starchy carbs, sugars, and alcohol... all contribute to a poor microbiome.

Note: Bad bacteria overgrowth, or what is called Candida overgrowth, does not look the same for every individual. You may relate to some of my symptoms, but not to others, and you may have your own unique symptoms. The list is quite long of signs of Candida overgrowth.

Balancing the gut is the key to relieving menstruated pain, as well as quieting sugar cravings in clearing up acne. I would not find this out until much later. I see that seventh grade girl in my memory and I wish I could give her the education then that did not come for fifteen more years!

My Health Part 3: *Thyroid/Hashimoto's*
Complete with body temperature issues (I dreaded being cold and always was), brittle nails, weight fluctuation, etc.

Quick recap:

Part 1 = Migraines

Part 2 = Acne, painful periods, and sugar cravings

Now... Part 3 - Diagnosis in my early 20s of Thyroid Disease/Hashimoto's Thyroiditis

As you can tell by now, I am such a diligent medical patient, and in my early 20s, at a routine annual physical, I was told that my thyroid seemed enlarged and I would have to take a series of tests. Sure enough, I was diagnosed with thyroid disease, as well as a thyroid full of nodules. One of the tests was an ultrasound guided needle biopsy of the nodules, one of the most painful tests I've experienced (no anesthesia, and a doctor with zero bedside manor = lame).

This is how it happened... Autoimmune disease occurs when the immune system makes antibodies against its own tissues (example is Hashimoto's Thyroiditis where the body makes antibodies to the thyroid gland). Studies have shown that gut imbalance can play a role in the development of autoimmune diseases like Hashimoto's Thyroiditis. As gut health declines, autoimmune disease gets worse.

The thyroid is an organ that produces hormones, and we all know by now that insulin is our dominant hormone. So when you balance your blood sugar, therefore balancing insulin, all other hormones fall into balance. Likewise, when blood sugar is out of balance, insulin is out of balance, and all other hormones follow suit.

Again, I had no idea that my symptoms were related at all! But look at all this... migraines, acne, sugar/soda cravings, painful periods... my body was trying to tell me something! My body was screaming at me that my gut health and blood sugars were gravely out of whack. And because I wasn't addressing it (I didn't know!)... the next symptom showed up - enter Hashimoto's!

Guys, in a span of ten years I am now on my fourth major symptom... and my fourth medical specialist, and I was only 23!... I'm young... way too young for so many prescriptions.

When I learned over a decade later, and then took the time to balance my gut and balance my blood sugar, I began to see a reversal in my thyroid symptoms. It is very slow and steady, but I was told by a top endocrinologist in Washington DC that I would never see a reversal of my thyroid disease symptoms. Other doctors told me that was not true at all. So I chose to believe them, and they have been right.

My Health Part 4: *Endometriosis*
Recap
Part 1 = migraines (age 13+)
Part 2 = painful periods, cystic acne, intense sugar cravings (age 19+)
Part 3 = thyroid disease (age 22+)
Now let's talk about endometriosis. Endometriosis is when the endometrial cells grow and bleed on the outside of the uterus each month, not just the inside. Many of the surrounding organs and tissues are also implanted with these cells (pelvis, bladder, ovaries, and others). And once all of these cells bleed, swelling starts, inflammation, and the immune system then kicks in its response.

In the 2002 study published in The Journal of Human Reproduction, it was shown that intestinal inflammation occurs more frequently in those with endometriosis than in those without. It also demonstrated that an inflamed gastrointestinal tract contains different microorganisms than a healthy gastrointestinal tract. Further, when there is gastrointestinal inflammation, Candida is especially prevalent. Simply said, endometriosis promotes further Candida growth. Later research discovered that endometriosis is directly associated with that inflammation, leaving women at even greater risk for toxic Candida overgrowth in the digestive tract.

Remember that Candida actually belongs in the human body and is meant to be a healthy part of a balanced inner ecosystem. Only when it grows beyond control does it pose a toxic threat. What causes it to grow beyond control? Poor diet and antibiotic use to name two.

Well that is what I was dealing with, symptoms of horrific pelvic pain, constipation, and later, severe unexplained infertility.

And until my mid 30s I was told by every doctor I saw that there was no cure for endometriosis, only pain management. Here we have another prescription, now for strong muscle relaxers and intense pain killers, which, by the way, also cause Candida overgrowth. The very drugs I took to get me through the pain of each month were only exacerbating future pain indefinitely.

If I only knew then what I know now. If I had only received the relief and healing that I have now... But then again, a part of me is so grateful for that experience because there is so much learning and helping and sharing that I can now pay forward.

Next up... Candida overgrowth left untreated reared its ugly head in the form of unexplained infertility.

My Health Part 5: Infertility
Recap
Part 1 = Migraines
Part 2 = Painful periods, acne, sugar cravings
Part 3 = Thyroid disease
Part 4 = Endometriosis
You would think that painful periods and endometriosis would be obvious indicators that I would have infertility. I

really did not know. I also married late – age 35 – so I didn't try to conceive until then.

I was optimistic to say the least – when I was not pregnant on month ONE after my wedding I was literally in tears because I was convinced it would happen quickly, and I had wanted children so badly. Well, one month was nothin'... we actually had years and years of fertility treatments, fertility prescriptions, artificial insemination, ultrasounds, surgery's, miscarriages that I stopped counting, and IVF. Nothing worked. Nothing. After 4 years we moved toward adoption.

Dare I say now that I am grateful for that period of infertility? I actually am, because nothing makes you take a more serious look at your health like your body not functioning correctly does... I began to delve and learn and study and pray like I never had before. I went to an acupuncturist... a seasoned Chinese man who was so wise and answered my countless questions. When typical Western medicine MD's simply told me I had 'unexplained infertility' and that I had a less-than-1% chance of conceiving, I went to other doctors who taught me about healing from the inside out. I learned about my blood sugar, and why the word 'glucose' kept coming up for me over the years in lab results, but not enough for a doctor to do anything about.

Here are some things I learned... fertility related gut issues that I had not known were linked:

PCOS
Endometriosis
Dysmenorrhea
Thyroid Problems
Adenomyosis
Estrogen dominance (estrogen is pro-inflammatory)
Autoimmune related infertility
Yeast infection
Pelvic inflammatory disease

I had several of those listed above – 5 to be exact. I learned that gut issues cause inflammation, and chronic inflammation around the gut leads to infertility. Infertility correlates with increased systemic inflammation, as well as pregnancy complications. I read that several studies show how probiotic supplementation reduces inflammation, demonstrating that it is plausible that use of probiotics reduce inflammation and enhance fertility.

Further, infections within any system can be incredibly detrimental to fertility. Our immune system is primarily in our gut, and when we have bad-bacteria overgrowth, our immune system is compromised, taking our fertility down along with it.

That is only the gut health part – blood sugar also correlates with fertility, as we already know that insulin is our dominant hormone – and hormone balance is critical for conception. Now all those lab results that were suggesting abnormal glucose levels were finally all tying in.

You want to all know how this story ends – I healed my gut and balanced my blood sugar and reduced my inflammation... slowly and steadily, and permanently. I had my first baby at 39 and my second baby at 44, after being told (quite sternly by a blunt fertility specialist) that I would never conceive. My symptoms of early menopause literally stopped. My painful periods stopped, along with my acne, and a slew of other ailments that I had walked around with for decades. You will never, ever, be able to convince me that balancing my three ROOT causes did not completely reverse my life, my health, and my ability to grow my family.

My Health Part 6: *Needing a Nap/Caffeine/Sleep*
Now I want to talk about sleep...
Sleep was always such a big deal to me. When I slept, I slept deeply, meaning I CRASHED. BUT, if I awakened for any reason (a phone call or a run to the bathroom), then returning

to sleep was impossible. I would lay there and lay there, and wait and wait to fall back to sleep. It was so frustrating. I would count the hours of rest that I was now losing, painfully aware of how tired I would be the next day. It was so confusing - how I could sleep so deeply but not return to sleep if it was interrupted. If I had to go to the bathroom in the night, I used to keep all of the lights off and get it over with quickly and try to not think or become alert in any way.

In the afternoons I would fight fatigue... oh would I fight fatigue (enter in sugar or soda to get me through). I had to arrange things just perfectly... meaning, I had to keep myself awake until bedtime so that I could truly fall asleep. I had to do all that I could to hear no interruptions that would wake me (as if I could control a fire engine driving down the street at night...) and when life would simply happen and I would be awakened, it would start all over again.

Then there was my need for a nap... when I would cave in and take the nap, you would think I had won the lottery it was such a big deal to me. I just could not imagine that anyone stayed awake all day and slept well at night and did not need a nap in between, or had to take stimulants. It was foreign to me that people could actually be awake for a full stretch of 16-18 hours and be energetic and happy and in good moods.

And let's talk about caffeine for a second... caffeine may be a Band-Aid... it may get you through to the end of the day and may be that necessary evil that we have all had to rely upon from time to time, but it is a TERRIBLE form of energy! It is jittery... it spikes and crashes... and it's addictive. It messes with your sleep rhythms, and it messes with your gut. It perpetuates the very problem it is trying to solve – fatigue!! Meaning, you may be getting-through-the-day, but you are actually making your REAL issues (as to why you have no energy in the first place) even worse and making you sicker.

Spoiler: When we get to the part where we can fast-forward about ten more years, you will see that I now never take naps, have sustained energy all day (not fake energy – literally NO caffeine or stimulants), even if I am up in the night with my little kids! Even then I am alert, look rested, am bright-eyed (no dark circles) happy, and I am present and there for my kids and my family. It is a whole new life... you cannot make this stuff up. When you are healthy – when you heal from the inside – everything changes.

Sleep is such a big deal – energy and rest are probably the number one issue I hear about from people... and also the number one SOLUTION that people are so happy about once they take charge of their health and fix it! We shout it from the rooftops because we almost cannot believe it is for real!!

Fecal Transplants

Have you ever heard of a fecal transplantation? Me neither...

Fecal microbiota transplant (FMT), also known as a stool transplant is a way to fight gut infection. Yes, it is a real thing and yes it is what you think it is. A fecal transplant involves inserting stool from a healthy donor into an unhealthy person's digestive tract to treat reoccurring infections. If you have tried other options with no success this may be something to learn more about.

Clostridium difficile infection can cause inflammation in the colon leading to diarrhea, cramping, and fever. People with Clostridium are given antibiotics to try to treat the infection. However, there are a certain number of patients that infection continues to come back after days and weeks of treatment. These patients have an increased risk of reoccurring infection and that is when a fecal transplant may be considered.

The desired result from the fecal transplant is to re-populate good bacteria in the gut that was destroyed present it is harder for infection to flourish and take hold. Fecal matter is not an ideal treatment to think about but the fecal matter has a variety of helpful bacteria, viruses, fungi and other organisms. This may be an option for someone that has tried all other avenues first.

A fecal transplant can be administered by a pill (yep, full of poop) that is swallowed by the patient. It can also be administered by inserting tubes going down the nose and into the stomach or small intestine to deposit the stool. More common a fecal transplant is administered during a colonoscopy. During a colonoscopy the colonoscope is advanced through the entire colon, as the colonoscope is pulled out it deposits the donor stool along the way. The length of time the patient holds on to the stool from the donor the more healthy bacteria from that stool is absorbed.

A review of existing research in the July 12, 2016, *PLOS Biology* suggests fecal transplants cure about 90% to 95% of cases of stubborn Clostridium difficile colitis. Fecal transplants are not yet covered by most insurance companies. Some insurance companies will cover this procedure if proven necessary. Donors of poop may receive a small amount for their poop donations for fecal transplants. Hopefully in the future it can become something that is more mainstreamed to solve health issues. If anything, we can learn more from this about how the benefits of healthy bacteria can restore gut health.

Secret 15

What Poor Gut Health Costs

Poor gut health has cost me years of missed enjoyment. Happiness I cannot get back. I experienced misery spending every spring and summer stuffed up with allergies, not being able to breathe without a nasal spray, eye drops, medications, and sleeping upright at night so I could breathe.

Years that I was constantly falling asleep while driving my kids to and from their activities, smacking my face and drinking water to stay awake and not crash the car.

It cost me losing handfuls of hair every day, stress from craving sugar uncontrollably, not feeling like I was in control of my food, but my food controlled me. Food was an enemy not a source of nutrition. It cost me time from always forgetting what I was doing (brain fog) and putting milk in the cupboard and cereal in the fridge.

It cost me happiness that I missed from being exhausted and losing the desire to live, having a black cloud that followed me around everywhere I went, always feeling like I was in a rut and needing to get out.

It cost me family time from wondering what life would be like for my husband and children when I was not around. Knowing I loved them so much, but I hated myself for not being able to be happy every day. I had no explained reason to feel helpless and lonely, I was surrounded by blessings and loved ones and I could not shake the depression and anxiety that consumed me. Feeling hopeless when it came to losing weight, knowing that even if I starved myself and exercised non-stop I still gained weight just by looking at a scale. Falsely thinking I needed to just accept my health. Hating my body and not trying to love it.

For others with poor health it cost them miscarriages, an inability to lose weight despite exercise and eating right. It cost them happiness for lost time spent sick or depressed. It cost them unwanted stress from diets that never worked, depression, anxiety, constipation, IBS issues, years and years of frustration trying to figure out what was wrong with their bodies and not knowing how to start feeling better again. It cost them time from wondering why they had a mystery pain or inflammation in their body. Why they had auto immune issues, mood, and hormone imbalances. They had sluggish and unmotivated feelings, feeling lethargic, premature aging, pale skin, acne or adult acne. They were chronically exhausted, have unexplained diarrhea, lactose intolerance, gluten intolerance, and more. All of these are ways poor gut health cost people when they do not know where to find the answers.

I do not want another person loosing precious time with family, friends, and happiness because they struggle with health issues. I want to shout from the rooftops what I have learned from my gut health secrets, so I can help others on their healing health journey. I share my research on gut health and what helped me in getting to the root cause of health issues in hopes that I may be able to help someone else that is out there searching for answers and not knowing where to look.

I want to help someone that has already tried everything they can think of, and the person who has just begun their journey into looking for answers. I am here to help You! I hope these gut health secrets have guided you in understanding gut health, how knowledge on gut health has evolved over the years and the new direction of proper gut health and how to achieve it. These secrets will not be secrets any longer.

Leah is a mom of four girls and one boy. Leah is originally from Northern California and now lives in San Antonio. Leah has a degree in Liberal Studies, a minor in Special Education, and now works at home teaching piano and voice lessons. Leah finally realized it was time to take charge and do something in her life to feel better; she gives hope to others that are wondering what to do now. Poor gut health cost Leah years of struggling and looking for answers. She is now ready to share what she has gained back after improving her health.

I think it is time to share my results from taking gut health supplements. I started taking probiotics and vitamins thirteen days ago. I decided to take them for two reasons-to increase my breast milk supply for my last baby and to get rid of my eczema!

I had been told by several friends and family members that the only way to truly get rid of eczema was to heal the gut and I had researched probiotics and felt good about the probiotics and vitamins being the answer to my gut health.

What I did not expect were the unexpected results that I saw right away. I am thirty-six weeks pregnant. My pregnancies are not easy by any means and by the end of them I can barely walk due to sciatic pain and general muscle soreness.

I am also very fatigued and have a hard time thinking when I am pregnant. This may be hard to believe (I probably would not believe it if I did not experience it) but the day after I started taking gut health supplements my soreness was gone.

I could easily get out of bed, I could pick something up off the floor without holding my breath because of the pain, I could play with my girls on the floor and then be able to get up off the floor easily.

I also had more energy! I am not feeling like I am going to pass out halfway through the day. I am so much happier and patient with my family because I am not so tired and cranky all the time.

I also noticed that my need/cravings for sugar were dramatically decreasing. Every day the cravings seem to go away a little more. I also am not as hungry all the time. My OBGYN told me that I did not need to gain any weight this pregnancy. I already had plenty of extra weight but I was struggling with that because I always felt like I was starving and if I was not constantly eating I would feel nauseous and I was gaining weight way too fast.

Since starting my probiotics and vitamins my weight has stabilized and I am not eating as much. Do not worry, I am still eating plenty just not overeating.

My eczema is still here but it definitely looks like it is healing. Fewer flare ups is a sign to me that it is getting better each day. When I have flareups I use my amazing microbiome skin cream to help clear it up. I am just so thankful for supplements that are helping me so much!

Secret 16

Now What?

You have been given a lot of information on gut health. You can take this information and apply it in your life and start feeling better.

You could also take this information and put it back on the shelf and wait for the day that you finally decide you need a change.

It is up to you, no one can make your life better except YOU!

I can buy you all the best food and supplements in the world, but you have to put them in your mouth. You have to have the discipline to drink the water your body needs. You have to decide to take a stand and know you are worth it. You have to decide and know that you are worthy of taking care of yourself and you can feel great again.

What are you going to do? Waiting only keeps you on the same path doing the same thing, and look at how that is going for you right now? If it was great you would not be reading this book.

Gut health is the key to feeling good, gut health is the key to a better future of living life to the fullest. When you have a proper balance of bacteria in your gut you will have the energy, strength and mental clarity to stay healthy and thrive. You can live your life to the fullest. You can be happy and have hope in the future.

Taking what you have learned and putting it into practice will take some time, and patience. Little by little you can make changes that will turn into bigger ones and then one day you will realize you are starting to feel better and you will like it.

If you are reading this book, I know you can do it!

Other Great Resources

Meyer, Emeran. *The Mind-Gut Connection*. New York: HarperCollins, 2016

Sonnenburg, Justin, Erica Sonnenburg. *The Good Gut*. New York: Penguin Press, 2015

Huffnagle, Gary B. *The Probiotic Revolution*. New york: Bantom, 2007

Sorokie, Alyce M. *Gut Wisdom*. Frankilin Lakes: Career Press, 2004

Kellman, Raphael. *The Microbiome Diet*. Boston: Da Capo Press, 2014

Thompson, Rob. *The Sugar Blockers Diet*. New York: Rodale, 2012

Thompson, Rob. *The Glycemic Load Diet*. New York: Rodale, 2012

Wentz, Izabells. *Hashimoto's Thyroiditis*. Chicago: Wentz LLC, 2013

Hyman, Mark. *The Blood Sugar Solution 10-Day Detox Diet*. New York: Little, Brown and Company, 2014

Flemin, Richard M. *Stop Inflammation Now!* New York: G.P. Putnam's Sons, 2004

Vaccariello, Liz. *Flat Belly Diet*. New York: Rodale, 2010

Glassman, Keri, Sarah Mahoney. *Slim Calm Sexy Diet*. New York: Rodale, 2012

Bhatia, Dr Tasneem. *21 Day Belly Fix*. Zinc Ink, September 23, 2014

Perlmutter, David. *Brainmaker.* Little, Brown Spark, April 28, 2015

Chutkan, Dr. Robynne *The Microbiome Solution* Avery, August 9, 2016

Romm, Aviva. *The Adrenal Thyroid Revolution.* HarperOne, January 31, 2017

Mullin, Gerard E. *The Gut Balance Revolution.* Rodale Books, July 3, 2017

About the Author

Rachel Miner was born an Entrepreneur. Daughter of a Dutch immigrant who lived the American Dream and taught her that anything is possible. She grew up playing "the money game" with her nine siblings learning how to create and run businesses in their home for days on end.

By age 12, she was braiding and styling hair for her friends, many of them arriving at 5am to 'get in' before school started. At the age of 14, Rachel started designing and sewing clothing for the mothers of the children she babysat. She taught Fiber Art classes for the local college and 4-H programs. This taste of having her own business sparked her interest to enter beauty school during her junior year of high school. She helped to support herself at this time by teaching sewing classes and making wedding dresses.

She successfully used her cosmetology degree to support herself through college, obtaining a BS degree in Business Management with an emphasis in International Business, Small Business, and Corporate Wellness.

Rachel owned and operated Sarah Jane's. Sarah Jane's was a full-service salon where half of the salon was actually a home decor store with items, gifts and accessories. While the ladies' hair was in process they could shop, redecorate their homes, and browse the latest and greatest knick knack bric-a-brac.

For years Rachel traveled around teaching people in the cosmetology industry how to be successful on the business side of beauty. Everything from choosing to be the best employee, booth renting or owning your own Salon and loving the choice your made.

Rachel has been in the health and wellness industry for over 30 years. She and husband, Shaun, have owned several businesses consisting of a health and full-service beauty salon, home decor, wedding consulting, a chain of dry cleaners and delivery service, a publishing company, real estate investing and consulting company, and a health and wellness company. They are the proud parents of seven children and continue to help people improve their lives every day.

Other great books by the author:

Beyond Beauty – Cosmetology Business Information and Resources. SJS Publishing 2003

How Foot Zoners Can Double Their Income This Year. SJS Publishing 2018

To learn more about Rachel go to HealAndBeHealthy.com

172

Acknowledgments

I wish to acknowledge my husband Shaun Miner who patiently stands beside me through all my crazy. He supports and loves me for who I am. He helps me with all my business adventures and generates all of the marketing, artwork and advertising for everything we do. I could not do what I do, without Shaun.

I want to thank Janie Van Komen, my mom, who edits many of my errors, gives encouragement, and inspiration to all my ideas. She inspires me with her love of writing. Even as a child she helped bring out my creative side. We made and sold all sorts of things from doll assessories to hand stitched teddy bear ornaments. She showed me to follow my Entrepreneur passions.

I want to thank all of my friends who shared stories, testimonials, advice and love in supporting me and helping me through my dream of writing this book. I love my lifelong friends who are now part of my One Big Happy Ohana.

I want to thank my Heavenly Father who gave me trials in my life to overcome and learn from so I can take that knowledge go out and help others.